£19.99

C

BW

Cari

Mer

Caring for Adults with Mental Health Problems

Edited by
I. PEATE
University of Hertfordshire

S. CHELVANAYAGAM
University of Hertfordshire

John Wiley & Sons, Ltd

Other Wiley Editorial Offices

John Wiley & Sons Inc., 111 River Street, Hoboken, NJ 07030, USA

Jossey-Bass, 989 Market Street, San Francisco, CA 94103-1741, USA

Wiley-VCH Verlag GmbH, Boschstr. 12, D-69469 Weinheim, Germany

John Wiley & Sons Australia Ltd, 42 McDougall Street, Milton, Queensland 4064, Australia

John Wiley & Sons (Asia) Pte Ltd, 2 Clementi Loop #02-01, Jin Xing Distripark, Singapore 129809

John Wiley & Sons Canada Ltd, 6045 Freemont Blvd, Mississauga, ONT, L5R 4J3

Wiley also publishes its books in a variety of electronic formats. Some content that appears in print may not
be available in electronic books.

Library of Congress Cataloging in Publication Data

Caring for adults with mental health problems / edited by Ian
  Peate, Sonya Chelvanayagam.
     p. ; cm.
  Includes bibliographical references and index.
  ISBN-13: 978-0-470-02629-8 (alk. paper)
  ISBN-10: 0-470-02629-4 (alk. paper)
  1. Psychiatric nursing. 2. Mental health services. I. Peate, Ian.
  II. Chelvanayagam, Sonya.
  [DNLM: 1. Mental Disorders. 2. Mental Health Services. WM 140 L438 2006]
  RC440.L43 2006
  616.89′0231—dc22
                                                            2006020143

British Library Cataloguing in Publication Data

A catalogue record for this book is available from the British Library

ISBN-13: 978-0470-02629-8
ISBN-10: 0-470-02629-4

Typeset in 10/12pt Times by Integra Software Services Pvt. Ltd, Pondicherry, India
Printed and bound in Great Britain by TJ International Ltd, Padstow, Cornwall
This book is printed on acid-free paper responsibly manufactured from sustainable forestry
in which at least two trees are planted for each one used for paper production.

Contents

Contributors

Thomas Beary, Senior Lecturer in Adult and Mental Health Nursing
BSc (Hons) Dip HE RN (Adult) RMN ENB Higher Award Advanced
Diploma in the Nursing Care of Older People
Thomas qualified as a Registered Mental Health Nurse in 1991 and worked in old age psychiatry in dementia care until 1994. He then worked as a Senior Staff Nurse and Junior Charge Nurse on the acute admission elderly psychiatry unit at Royal Free Hospital. In 1995, Thomas was promoted to Senior Charge Nurse in old age psychiatric rehabilitation. In 1999, he trained as an RN (Adult) with Middlesex University. Thomas's previous position was as a discharge nurse coordinator with Watford and Three Rivers Primary Care Trust based at West Hertfordshire Hospitals NHS Trust.

Alan Brownbill, Senior Lecturer in Mental Health
BSc (Hons) Microbiology PGCE RN Dip Counselling
Alan started mental health nursing in 1977 in Somerset. Prior to becoming a Nurse Tutor and Lecturer, he worked in psychiatric day hospitals taking a particular interest in counselling and therapeutic relationships. Alan has been Module Leader for courses in therapeutic interventions and mental health promotion. He is currently developing work in supporting people who are bereaved, with counselling.

Sonya Chelvanayagam, Senior Lecturer in Mental Health
MSc PgDip (Learning and Teaching) RN
Sonya qualified as a Mental Health Nurse in 1985. She then trained as a Registered General Nurse. Sonya has worked in a range of different settings caring for individuals with a combination of physical symptoms and mental health problems. Most notably, she developed a mental health nurse service within a specialist mental health team for people attending HIV/GUM services. Sonya works as a Senior Lecturer in mental health at the University of Hertfordshire and as a Lecturer in the Burdett Institute of Gastrointestinal Nursing, King's College London.

Stephen John Cloudsdale
RMN RGN BA (Hons) PostGrad Dip PGCE ILTM
Stephen is a Senior Lecturer in Mental Health at the University of Hertfordshire. His clinical experience has included working with those with drug problems and providing day services for mentally ill people within the community. He has been a

Senior Lecturer for over 12 years and has an interest in the history of mental health care and ethics.

Angela Edmonds, Senior Occupational Therapist
Dip COT

Angela has worked in mental health services for 22 years across a range of areas, and for the past 18 years in community mental health services. Angela's specialist interests are in group work and anxiety management using a cognitive behavioural approach.

Sue Hahn, Senior Lecturer in Mental Health
MA Gerontology RMN PGCE

Sue trained as an RMN and is currently a Senior Lecturer in Mental Health at the University of Hertfordshire. She has worked as a Research and Training Officer and a Community Mental Health Nurse for people with dementia and their families, and Community Mental Health Nurse with people with substance misuse problems.

Clare Hubbard, Drama Therapist
BA (Hons) in Theatre and Media Drama MA in Dramatherapy

Clare works as a Dramatherapist with adults with mental health problems in Hertfordshire Partnership NHS Trust. Clare completed her initial degree in Theatre and Media Drama in 1995. She qualified as a Dramatherapist in 1998 and completed her Master's in 2003, both at the University of Hertfordshire. Her dissertation was on *The Dramatherapy Group on the Acute Psychiatric Ward*. Currently, Clare is an Executive Officer of the British Association of Dramatherapists and chair of its NHS subcommittee. Before qualifying, Clare worked for some years as a Residential Support Worker with adults with learning disabilities.

Paul Illingworth, Academic/Professional Lead Mental Health
MA BSc (Hons) Dip N PGCE RN RPHEA

Paul began adult nursing in 1974, and then moved to mental health in 1979, since when he has spent the rest of his career in clinical, operational and strategic management positions. Paul has nearly 20 years' teaching experience at both pre- and post-qualification levels. Paul's teaching has involved the education of psychologists, social workers, physiotherapists, doctors, midwives, and paramedics as well as nurses. Additionally, he has undertaken consultancy work for Her Majesty's Prison Service College for England and Wales.

Soo Lee, Senior Lecturer in Mental Health
MSc (Lond) PgDip Mental Health Work PgCert (Learning and Teaching)
RGN RMN

Soo has a background in mental health nursing and NHS management. She was a member of the Mental Health Act Commission and Code of Practice Review

Group. Currently, she serves as a member of the Mental Health Review Tribunal. She writes on and is an active researcher in mental health practice. Soo is a Senior Lecturer at the University of Hertfordshire, and leads postgraduate programmes in mental health studies. She has just completed a major research study into the subject of physical restraint.

Yvonne Mitchell, Senior Lecturer in Mental Health
BEd (Hons) ILTM RNT RMN RGN SEN (Scotland)

Yvonne completed her nurse education as an Enrolled Nurse in Glasgow in 1982. She moved to Hertfordshire and, returning to studies, she completed her RMN (1985) and subsequent RGN in Bedfordshire (1987). She became manager of a Regional Brain Injury Unit on returning to Hertfordshire and completed the Diploma in Nursing Studies. Subsequently, this led her into education, completing the B.Ed (Hons) at Sussex University in 1989. Academically her interests are women's issues and Schizophrenia and their impact on family dynamics.

Ian Peate, Associate Head of School
EN (G) RGN DipN (Lond) RNT BEd (Hons) MA (Lond) LLM

Ian began his nursing career in 1981 at Central Middlesex Hospital, becoming an Enrolled Nurse working in an intensive care unit. He later undertook three years' student nurse training at Central Middlesex and Northwick Park Hospitals, becoming a Staff Nurse then a Charge Nurse. He has worked in nurse education since 1989. His key areas of interest are nursing practice and theory, sexual health and HIV/AIDS. He is currently Associate Head of School. His portfolio centres on recruitment and marketing and professional academic development within the School of Nursing and Midwifery.

Brian Thomson, Senior Lecturer in Mental Health
MA RMN

Brian worked as a community psychiatric nurse and cognitive behavioural therapist for 20 years with a special interest inpersonality disorders. He currently lectures in mental health and cognitive behavioural therapy at the University of Hertfordshire.

Acknowledgements

We would like to thank all of our colleagues for their help, support, comments and suggestions. We would particularly like to thank the students on the Certificate in Community Mental Health Care Course September 2003 and September 2004 (West Herts College), who provided assistance and suggestions on subjects to be included in this text. We would also like to thank Viewpoint in Hertfordshire, service user training and education unit, for their feedback on the chapters.

Sonya would like to thank her husband Gavey and brother Martin Wood for their understanding and support.

Ian would like to thank his partner Jussi for all of his continued support and encouragement.

1 Introduction

I. PEATE AND S. CHELVANAYAGAM

Caring for Adults with Mental Health Problems aims to offer a foundation for those who provide, or wish to provide, health care and support for people with mental health problems. Those who have contributed to the book come from various backgrounds – both practice and academia. The authors are committed to creating and sustaining a positive mental health environment for all; they believe that each person is a unique being with individual needs and aspirations – each chapter of this book reflects these values, attitudes and hopes.

Caring for those who have mental health problems can be complex and rewarding; making a difference really does mean that. It is estimated that at least as many as one in six adults experiences mental ill health at some time in their life; furthermore, the World Health Organization predict that by 2020 depression will be the leading cause of disability (Collishaw *et al.* 2004). Those who have mental health problems can face discrimination and prejudice in society, for example they may have difficulty in accessing education and other statutory services as a result of their illness. There are some members of our society who are excluded from accessing services because of mental health legislation; Lee in her chapter concerning legal matters (Chapter Six) considers those individuals.

We wholeheartedly believe that people with mental health problems deserve the best possible care and support; in order to offer this, mental health professionals must have an understanding of the context of the individual service user's life, both in the community and also within the various healthcare settings. Those who are supported effectively in the community can remain well. This text is designed to encourage the reader to push forward the possibilities associated with mental health care, providing innovative and contemporary approaches to care and support. The notion of partnership is central to effective client-centred care. It is vital that care and support are to be delivered in the most appropriate manner, and this text encourages the reader to apply this approach to care delivery in any situation in which they may be working. In Illingworth's chapter (Chapter Four), the importance of partnership working and the benefits that this may bring the patient are emphasised, looking beyond a disease-orientated approach to one where the patient is central. Such an approach is in tandem with the current Government's

Caring for Adults with Mental Health Problems   Edited by I. Peate and S. Chelvanayagam
© 2006 John Wiley & Sons, Ltd

desire to provide a health service that is designed around the patient, as opposed to the needs of the patient being forced to fit around the service already provided (Department of Health 2006).

The primary audience for this text are nursing students, those who are undertaking NVQ/SNVQ, Access to Nursing, Cadet nursing programmes of study and those returning to practice, but not exclusively those cited. The text may feel as comfortable on the shelves of a book case at home as in an academic library. However, the text should not be seen as a comprehensive book discussing all the needs of the person with a mental health problem – that would be an impossibility – rather the reader is encouraged to identify further topics of importance that have not been considered here and to delve deeper. The terms and the philosophies applied to this book can be adapted to suit a number of health care workers at various levels and in a range of settings in order to develop individual health care workers' caring, informed skills.

The book uses up-to-date information that the reader will require in order to begin to understand how to help, support and care for those with mental health problems both in the institutional setting (e.g. the hospital) and in the community (e.g. the home setting). The material is organised in such a way that it reflects contemporary practice in a user-friendly manner; in addition, information is related to clinical practice issues that may be experienced when working with people with mental health problems, their families and friends. It is not envisaged that the text be read from cover to cover in one sitting; it has been designed to be used as a reference book (a resource, a reader) either in the clinical setting, classroom or at home.

The text should be seen as a handbook or a manual that has a sound evidence base, and one that will challenge and encourage the reader to develop a questioning approach to care provision. It emphasises the integration of theory and practice. If you are currently studying, in order to get the most out of this book you are strongly encouraged to attend all of your classes associated with your current programme of study, using this text to supplement and support your theoretical and clinical learning. Much of the discussion is placed against the backdrop of the Mental Health Act 1983 and *A National Service Framework for Mental Health* (Department of Health 1999). Other key documents, publications and statutes are also used to inform debate.

The overarching aims are to help the reader to understand the fundamental aspects of care in order to facilitate safe and effective practice; to stimulate thought and to generate discussion – this will encourage the development of effective caring skills underpinned by a sound knowledge base. This is a foundation text that will enable personal growth in relation to mental health care.

CHANGES IN SOCIETY

It is important to set the scene, putting into context the extent to which society lives and changes in an attempt to understand the needs of those who you may need to provide care and support for. The proportion of those who live alone is expected to increase over the next 20 years. This is due to several factors, for example an increased longevity, as well as changes in familial structures. Contemporary society is much more geographically mobile than it was 20 years ago. Twenty-one per cent of those aged 65 years or over see their family or friends less than once a week or not at all (Office of National Statistics 2001). The consequences of these changes can result in profound mental health problems and challenges, and will have an impact on the individual, their friends, carers and service providers.

MENTAL HEALTH ISSUES AND THE OLDER POPULATION

The number of those aged 65 years and over with mental health problems is growing. Those aged 65 years and over with mental health problems will rise in the next ten years by 10%, with the greatest burden being on those who are aged over 80 years. Depression and dementia are common problems that will increase in the elderly population (Department of Health 2005). Hahn in her chapter regarding the dementias (Chapter Thirteen) discusses these issues further.

A WORD ABOUT TERMINOLOGY

Often a difficult task when writing a textbook is the choice of the terms to be used. It is important to define terms from the outset as different terms can mean different things to different people. There are a diversity of terms that can be used to describe people with mental health problems. Using any term can lead to labelling; Brownbill in his chapter considers the implications associated with using labels in his discussion on contemporary views associated with mental health and mental illness (Chapter Three).

A common expression that is often used within the NHS is 'patient', and on a few occasions this has been used in this text. It is acknowledged that not everyone supports the use of the passive concept associated with this term; it can emphasise the medical focus of the relationship between the person and the service.

The use of 'client' can have the potential to emphasise the professional nature of the relationship. Client and consumer have their roots in health care provision during the 1980s and 1990s, when market forces and consumerism were to the fore.

More recently, the term 'expert' has been used, the emphasis being placed on a participative approach, which acknowledges a person's capacity to work towards their own rehabilitation. Experts are seen to be on a par with the experts who provide care, for example a nurse or doctor. This term values the views and experiences of the expert: the service user.

Not all people like the terms 'service user' or 'user'; such terminology could lead to the grouping together of an otherwise diverse community of individuals with very individual needs. The term 'user' may also have some negative connotations associated with it. It could be used to identify those who are involved in the use of illicit substances.

'People with mental health problems' is a term that has already been used in this introductory section. This is a broad definition that is often used by various agencies. In this context, it has the potential to acknowledge that many people can experience mental health problems and that those problems cannot necessarily be understood in terms of being an illness or a disease.

'Survivor' is a term that is relatively new and can be used to describe people who have experienced life events such as sexual abuse, torture, racism or sexual oppression. When used appropriately, it can empower the person. Often the term is used by self-help groups and other voluntary organisations.

This text uses various terms and aims to promote the care and support of those with mental health difficulties and mental health distress. The terms used here cover a wide range of experiences that may affect anyone at any time. There are many terms, which should be avoided, that will only result in stigma and prejudice, causal words such as 'mad' or 'crazy' must be avoided at all times. Try to listen to and respect the terminology that is being used by those who are experiencing mental health difficulties themselves.

The phrase 'carer' has been used on many occasions in this book. This term is used to describe those who look after others, whether they be ill, healthy or have a disability. 'Carer' has many interpretations and may refer to a professional health care worker or to an unpaid relative, friend or volunteer providing care. It has been estimated that there are approximately six million unpaid carers in the UK (Carers UK 2005); this figure includes parents, grandparents and siblings who are looking after sick children.

THE CHAPTERS

It has already been stated that this text does not attempt to address every aspect of mental health care. The chapters have been arranged in order to provide insight into the complexities of providing care to those who may have a mental health problem. This book endeavours to provide the reader with a straightforward understanding of some of the issues that may impinge on an individual's well-being.

Chapter Two sets the scene and places mental health care in an historical context. The history of mental health care is brought up to date with a discussion of contemporary philosophies and ways of understanding the complex phenomena associated with mental health and mental health illness. Chapter Three considers the various perspectives regarding mental illness. The chapter includes a discussion of the models of mental health care that can be used and also the effects these may have on an individual's well-being.

Chapter Four considers the importance of partnership working within mental health care. The health care worker never operates in isolation, he or she is a part of a multidisciplinary team, and effective communication within this team is vital if the best quality care is to be provided. Caring for the person with mental health problems can sometimes be challenging, and those working in the mental health arena must liaise with a range of health and social care professionals from various statutory, independent and voluntary agencies. Those health and social care professionals and their roles are described.

Mental health promotion is primarily concerned with how individuals and communities can enhance and influence the mental health of the nation. Chapter Five identifies how emotional resilience can be enhanced to enable an individual's positive sense of well-being, promoting dignity and worth. Mental health promotion takes place in various settings, and the application of mental health promotion in some of these settings is discussed. Fulfilling an individual's health potential is central to care, and this chapter discusses various health-promotion strategies.

In Chapter Six, issues concerning the law, ethics and morals are discussed. Insight into some of the key statutory legislation that governs mental health care is provided. In addition, the chapter is designed to enhance the reader's understanding and knowledge of the legal ramifications of working with people with mental health problems in order that they may be able to confidently approach this work.

Chapters Seven to Thirteen provide the reader with insight and understanding associated with a number of common presenting mental health problems. These chapters also outline the potential interventions required. Generally, the aetiology, prevalence (if appropriate), presenting features, care and management of various mental health problems are outlined. Consideration has been taken to steer away from labelling as well as using a medical model approach. A holistic, individualised approach is advocated by the authors of these chapters.

Approaches associated with mental health care are described in Chapter Fourteen in an attempt to explain how carers can help the individual, a therapeutic/helping approach is advocated. The care planning process is outlined; effective communication and interpersonal skills are central to practice. The chapter explores various types of intervention – from medical interventions to psychotherapeutic ones and art therapies, such as dramatherapy and art therapy – as well as discussing the role of the service user's family.

We have endeavoured to provide you with an interesting, informative and up-to-date snapshot of mental health care. We have enjoyed this challenge and hope that you find the chapters interesting and thought-provoking, and, most importantly, we anticipate that the care and support you provide will be enhanced as a result of your learning.

REFERENCES

Carers UK (2005) *A Manifesto for Carers*. London, Carers UK.
Collishaw S, Maughan B, Goodman R, Pickles A (2004) *Time Trends in Adolescent Health*. London, Nuffield Foundation.
Department of Health (1999) *A National Service Framework for Mental Health*. London, Department of Health.

Department of Health (2005) *Independence, Well-being and Choice: Our Vision for the Future of Social Care for Adults in England.* London, Department of Health.

Department of Health (2006) *Our Health, Our Care, Our Say: A New Direction for Community Services.* London, Department of Health.

Office of National Statistics (2001) *Living in Britain: General Household Survey 2001.* London, The Stationery Office.

2 History of Mental Health Care

S. CLOUDSDALE

INTRODUCTION

This chapter aims to examine the history of approaches and change in attitudes towards those living with mental illness. It will examine the treatment based upon these approaches and will consider provision of care within societies over time. An historical account related to the elements of mental health care provision is also included.

The question that must be addressed is: 'Have attitudes to those living with a mental illness changed over time and has the treatment (from the general public as well as health care professionals) changed accordingly?' The change in attitude, from a harsh to a more accepting view of the plight of the mentally ill, dictated how those with mental illness were viewed and how they were treated. This is linked to what people regarded as being abnormal or mad in a given culture or at a given time. Attitudes change and values change with them; not many in Western society will care very much if people go about almost nude on the summer beaches; however, attitudes even 50 years ago would have been very different and most people would have been outraged with present-day behaviour. The important thing here is that society's views as to what is acceptable in relation to dress have changed and attitudes to what constitutes appropriateness of controlling dress codes will have changed also, and so it is with attitudes towards those living with mental health problems.

Society's attitudes towards those living with mental health problems are guided by the prevailing and accepted explanation for causes of such behaviour.

ANIMISM AND RELIGIOUS EXPLANATIONS

In primitive or pre-modern societies, the belief that everything has a 'soul' or 'spirit', even inanimate objects, is called 'animism'. Primitive people would have tried to explain the natural phenomena around them in terms of spirits acting upon the person and causing the events they were trying to explain. This explanation held for mental illness, or 'madness'. The explanation was that some form of spirit had taken possession of the afflicted person and was causing them to display the bizarre behaviour that was being witnessed (Rosenhan & Seligman 1995). The invading

Caring for Adults with Mental Health Problems   Edited by I. Peate and S. Chelvanayagam
© 2006 John Wiley & Sons, Ltd

spirit was viewed as being parasitic and was to be removed as any other parasite. Some of the physical interventions included the use of 'trephines', where holes were made in the skulls of affected people to enable the 'spirits' to leave the body of the person.

The belief was that people could be possessed by all manner of spirits: those of ancestors, animals, gods or those that the person had wronged. The view was that the person may or may not be to blame for the position they were in; and the services of helpers such as shamans or witch doctors were necessary to alleviate the symptoms of the demonic possession and ultimately to expel the unwelcome spirit (Douglas 1970). It is important to note that the bizarre behaviour sometimes demonstrated was tolerated within limits. A reason for this may be that madness was an example of what the gods could do to you and so the common view was 'who are we to punish you further?' It was also the case that many people resorted to sorcerers and witches to procure potions and spells. The classical world institutionalised sooth-saying and oracles in the form of temple religion with a pantheon of gods. The intervention of these gods was seen as the main explanation for the symptoms of madness; moreover, these symptoms, such as hearing voices, were seen as evidence of divine favour in some societies, and the affected person would have found a role that was valued by that society.

With the advent of Christianity, the position of the mad within society deteriorated. The Church would allow no avenue into the supernatural world other than by its own strictly controlled rites, and any person who seemed to possess an illegitimate and special insight into the beyond (some mentally ill people seemed to be in this category) was to be condemned as being influenced by demonic forces (Ellenberger 1970).

The rise in the view that the mentally ill were demonically controlled coincided with terrible upheavals within the Church in the sixteenth century. The Protestant reformation was a disruption that smashed the social equilibrium that had prevailed for centuries (Trevor-Roper 1970). It was within this disrupted context that the belief in the malign influence of witches flourished. The Church had considered witchcraft to be an 'illusion' at one time, but now it was viewed as a heresy and punishable by death. There were handbooks to help the religious authorities find these witches; the most famous is *Malleus Maleficarum*, which means 'hammer of the witches', which was published in the late fifteenth century by two Dominican monks, Sprenger and Kramer (Summers 1971). This document helped the religious authorities persecute thousands of people, mostly women, who did not fit into the changing structures of European society.

The mentally ill were especially vulnerable, largely because their experiences were in some cases quite bizarre and unintelligible to those investigating them. If asked if they thought they were hearing voices from another world, the person would probably answer 'yes' and thus condemn themselves.

A conservative estimate is that from the fifteenth to the seventeenth centuries about 100,000 people, mostly women, in Europe and in the American colonies were put to death as a result of this persecution (Deutsch 1949). How many of these people were mentally ill, it is impossible to know with any accuracy; however, it must be remembered that it was not normal behaviour that brought these people to the attention of the authorities.

As was stated at the beginning of this chapter, the treatment that the mentally ill received was dependent on the prevailing view regarding its causation. Those who were thought to be possessed by demons underwent various forms of exorcism, where these spirits were supposed to be driven from the body of the victim. If this was unsuccessful, casting the person out of society or ostracism was the next step. However, once the affected person was in this position they were vulnerable to the full terrors of the Church.

PHYSICAL EXPLANATIONS

Alongside the supernatural explanation for abnormal behaviour, there has been a long history concerning the physical causation of mental illness. The evidence concerning trephining in ancient Egypt is an example of how a physical intervention could help to alleviate mental distress, albeit from a supernatural cause. The most notable example of a physical cause being ascribed to a mental illness is contained in the explanation of hysteria. Early Greek physicians took the view that the epileptic-type seizures and complaints of anxiety, dizziness, paralysis, depression, blindness and physical disability were caused, in women, by a wandering uterus.

These physicians believed that the uterus could become detached from its usual place and move about all over the body. The uterus was thought to attach itself to places and organs in the body and thus affect the body's ability to function effectively. If the uterus were to attach itself to the liver, the woman would lose her voice; if it moved to the chest, it would cause convulsions and epilepsy (Rosenhan & Seligman 1995). This view held for many centuries; however, the Roman physician Galen (second century CE) alleged that the uterus was not an organ that wandered about the body like a separate animal but rather that it was a stationary sex organ that became inflamed, and that this was the cause of the symptoms of hysteria. Galen suggested that mental distress had a sexual origin in both women and men. He came to this conclusion after observing that both men and women suffered similar symptoms after sexual abstinence; the view that some mental distress has a sexual origin is one that has survived to this day (Veith 1965).

For the most part, physical explanations settled on an 'animalist' point of view. This maintained that because animals and some mad people were not in control of themselves there were similarities between them, and the most obvious similarity was that both lacked the power of 'reason'. This view allowed people to treat the mentally ill in much the same way as they treat animals, i.e. without restraint and cruelly. The mentally ill person could be kept in strict and miserable conditions:

> The ease with which certain of the insane of both sexes bear the most rigorous and prolonged cold... On certain days when the thermometer indicated... as many as 16 degrees below freezing a madman could not endure his wool blanket, and remained

sitting on the icy floor of his cell. In the morning, one no sooner opened his door than he ran in his shirt into the inner court, taking ice and snow by the fistful, applying it to his breast and letting it melt with a sort of delectation. (Foucault 1965)

The development of more modern medical approaches pointed to a more enlightened view of mental illness. The view developed, in the nineteenth century, that mental illness was a disease of the body and, therefore, could be treated as any other physical disease. Present-day pharmacology echoes this transition towards a more humane and medical model of treatment.

Most treatments for mental distress before the late eighteenth century, from a physical perspective, were based on the concept of the four humours:

- blood
- black bile
- phlegm
- yellow bile.

It was thought that these four fluids had to be in equilibrium to preserve a person's health, both physical and mental. If any one of these fluids predominated, the person would fall ill. The physician would seek to bring the person back into equilibrium by relieving the body of the excess fluid. This mostly involved bleeding the person by opening a vein or purging the person by administering either an emetic to make them vomit or an aperient (enema) to purge their body of impurities. The mentally ill were subjected to this form of treatment and it was found that those who were excitable or raging could be made calm by copious bleeding (Rosenhan & Seligman 1995). However, those who could not afford such physical treatment, the majority, were cared for by their families as best they could.

PSYCHOLOGICAL EXPLANATIONS

The ancient world had views on the psychological nature of the origin of some mental illnesses. Through observation, Galen found that thoughts alone could have an effect upon the body; for example he found that the pulse rate could be affected by thinking about emotionally charged situations – such as being in battle or thinking of one's lover. However, this approach was forgotten for centuries until it revived in the middle of the eighteenth century. One of the first to put forward a purely psychological interpretation of mental illness was Franz Anton Mesmer (1734–1815). Mesmer put forward the notion that many instances of mental distress could be explained by reference to 'universal magnetic fluid'. This 'fluid', which was invisible and impalpable, flowed through the human body. Its obstruction was the cause of the symptoms of hysteria, depression, anxiety and loss of reason. The universal magnetic fluid was later called 'animal magnetism'. Mesmer worked in Paris in the 1770s where he provided 'clinics'; at these clinics, people gathered around large wooden tubs that were full of water and magnetic iron filings. The assembled 'patients' would hold on to iron rods that were dipped into the fluid contained in the tubs. The iron rods were placed on various parts of the patient's body and the 'magnetic fluid' was supposed to be concentrated by this procedure and thus bring forth the patient's crisis. One by one, the patients would start to feel strange tingling sensations; this would lead to a general experience of convulsions and trembling.

Eventually, the authorities in Paris looked into the claims of Mesmer and declared them 'without foundation and fraudulent', declaring that his cures were effected by 'imagination'. Anton Mesmer was then not heard from again.

This was interesting in that many of those who took part in the 'cures' reported an alleviation or disappearance of their symptoms (Rosenhan & Seligman 1995). If this was the result of 'imagination', it could be argued that some of the mental distress experienced was also from the 'imagination'; by this is meant that the cause of the symptoms were psychological and not physical in origin: the symptoms themselves were real to the sufferer.

In the nineteenth century, the work of Jean-Martin Charcot (1825–1893) followed in the psychological tradition. His speciality was the nervous system, and distinguishing hysterical convulsions from epileptic seizures. In this pursuit he used hypnosis. He demonstrated that some people who reported paralysis in their limbs could move them under hypnosis. A diagnosis of 'hysteria' would be given in this case. However, modern thinking is that Charcot's students coached his patients to perform and that many of them were not hypnotised at all (Ellenberger 1970). However, in his clinic Charcot trained a large number of neurologists, one of whom was Sigmund Freud.

The treatment that the mentally ill would be offered from this perspective was one based on the concept of the 'unconscious'. This view held that there were psychological forces at work that the affected person had no direct knowledge of. Sigmund Freud (1856–1939) worked on a cathartic method that encouraged people to talk about their troubles under hypnosis. Freud eventually moved to a technique where he still encouraged the same sort of therapeutic disclosure but without using hypnosis – psychoanalysis (Phillips 2006).

PSYCHIATRIC HOSPITALS

The majority of those suffering from mental distress were not suitable for, or could not afford, the esoteric treatments of the psychodynamic practitioners. These people were subject to segregation from society. In the nineteenth century, the building of asylums for the mentally ill was undertaken in Britain. This form of large heavily populated institution located in the countryside was the norm until the 1970s and 1980s (Rothman 2002). After this time, the aim has been to empty these large institutions and to relocate those living with mental illness into the community. This move is related to the concept of 'care in the community'.

The story of the rise of the mental institution starts with the provision of accommodation for the poor and those begging in Paris in the early seventeenth century. The *Hôpital Général*, which included *La Salpêtrière* and *La Bicêtre*, were former Lazar houses, i.e. hospitals for those suffering from leprosy (Hansen's Disease). Leprosy, for the most part, disappeared from Europe at this time, leaving these large and financially endowed institutions with very few inmates. The decision was taken to place the poor and those begging into these institutions; at face value, this may appear to have been a humane thing to have done. However, the view of the public was that all these people were not gainfully employed and this was not because of economic conditions or bad luck on the part of the inmates; it was seen as being due to their individual moral failure and indolence. These institutions were easily converted into workhouses where the inmates were expected to work; however, the institution would pay them only a fraction of the going rate for such work conducted outside the institution (Foucault 1965). The mentally ill were soon segregated within these institutions and would receive very poor care, as well as being kept in unsanitary conditions, and were subjected to abuse by the warders.

This situation was much the same in London. In the St Mary of Bethlehem hospital (known as Bethlem or Bedlam), the mentally ill were incarcerated and chained to the walls. This sort of treatment looks incredibly cruel from our modern perspective, but it must be remembered that the prevailing view was that those who were mentally ill had lost their 'reason' and had degenerated to the level of an animal, that in some way they had lost their humanity. Therefore, these people had to be controlled in the same way as one controlled animals, i.e. with firmness and fear. This regime of control would include mechanical restraint and even physical assault (Scull 1981).

This 'cruel' approach was not universal. At the end of the eighteenth century, people such as Vincenzo Chiarugi (1759–1820) in Italy and Philippe Pinel (1745–1826) in France were put in charge of the institutions that housed the insane. They thought that the general bad treatment of the insane – close incarceration, chaining up and physical abuse – was the main reason for their violent and disruptive behaviour. They were not against 'coercion' in regard to these people but believed that this coercion should be psychological and not physical. Their method was one of unchaining the mentally ill and bringing them up from the underground chambers in which they were kept and into the light and fresh air (Foucault 1965).

A more humane or 'moral' approach was instituted in England at this period. William Tuke (1732–1822), a Quaker of York, set up the Retreat there in 1796. This place was to provide a quiet refuge for some of the insane. It was based on kindness, courtesy and dignity. It was not a lunatic asylum but a place where the inmates were treated as part of the family. The person coming in would be invited to dine with the family running it and was treated with respect. However, Tuke was adamant that the mentally ill person should control themselves and not let their symptoms get the better of them. In this way, the constraints applied to the mentally ill were no longer external but internal. The mentally ill had to behave themselves or else they could be excluded from the Retreat (Scull 1981).

In 1845, the County Asylums Act compelled every county and borough in England and Wales to provide asylum and treatment for its poor 'lunatics', as the term was, and in the same year the Lunacy Act set up a commission that had authority over all asylums. It was to monitor the erection of all public and private asylums. The 1890 Lunacy Act was a major consolidating Act that remained the core of English and Welsh lunacy legislation until the Mental Health Act 1959 (Scull 1981). This was superseded by the Mental Health Act 1983. The purpose of these Acts of Parliament was to regulate the treatment of the mentally ill and to provide them with much needed protection; they stated what was required to detain people against their will and what sort of mental illnesses could be treated without consent. Built into these Acts (especially the 1983 Act) were legal controls on the application of electroconvulsive therapy (ECT) as well as a system of review tribunals that had input from nurses to protect these vulnerable people (Lee & Cloudsdale 2000). Section 117 of the 1983 Mental Health Act imposes a duty on local services and health authorities to provide after-care for some mentally ill people. The situation at the time of writing is that we are awaiting a new Mental Health Act.

In 1999, the present Government brought in a National Service Framework (NSF) for mental health. The NSF is designed to offer mental health services that are set by the National Institute for Health and Clinical Excellence, delivered by clinical governance and monitored by the commission for health improvement. The aims of the NSF are to ensure a high-quality mental health service for the modern age (Department of Health, 1999); its main task is to set standards in five areas:

1. mental health promotion
2. primary care and access to services
3. effective services for people with severe mental illness
4. caring about carers
5. preventing suicide.

The overall aims of this policy are to promote mental health and to combat discrimination. It is designed to ensure that those with mental health problems have their needs assessed and are offered effective treatments. The policy also aims to support those who are caring for people with mental health problems and to bring down the incidence of suicide. This policy is a far cry from the attitudes of the nineteenth century and encourages care providers to deliver care that is humane and of high quality.

CONCLUSION

Changing views can result in changing approaches and practices. Those living with mental illness have been on the receiving end of attitudes and treatment that have been dictated by the changing views of what causes mental illness and how it should be treated; this gradual change in approach towards how the mentally ill are treated is still at work today.

Over time, there have been accepted ways of dealing with people with mental health problems and the care provided at that period in time was, however well intentioned, inhumane and punitive in approach. Enlightened approaches have and are beginning to emerge.

The new millennium sees mental health care as moving from a medically dominated model to a more social model of multidisciplinary mental health care with the individual at the centre of the model. Often, distress was seen as a response to biological disequilibrium; more and more the causes of mental distress are being seen in a broader context and the issues that have a profound effect on the person and society are slowly being addressed in a more holistic manner.

REFERENCES

Department of Health (1999) *National Service Framework for Mental Health: Modern Standards and Service Models*. London, The Stationery Office.

Deutsch A (1949) *The Mentally Ill in America*. New York, Columbia University Press.

Douglas M (1970) *Witchcraft: Confessions and Accusations*. London, Tavistock.

Ellenberger HE (1970) *The Discovery of the Unconscious: The History and Evolution of Dynamic Psychiatry*. New York, Basic Books.

Foucault M (1965) *Madness and Civilisation: A History of Insanity in an Age of Reason*. New York, Random House.

Lee SM, Cloudsdale SJ (2000) The nurse's role in mental health review tribunals. *Mental Health Practice* **4**(2): 10–12.

Phillips A (ed) (2006) *The Penguin Freud Reader*. London, Penguin.

Rosenhan DL, Seligman EP (1995) *Abnormal Psychology* (3rd edn.). London, WW Norton.

Rothman D (1971) *The Discovery of the Asylum: Social Order and Disorder in the New Republic*. New York, Walter de Gruyter.

Scull A (ed) (1981) *Madhouses, Mad-doctors and Madmen: The Social History of Psychiatry in the Victorian Age*. Philadelphia, University of Pennsylvania.

Summers M (1971) *Witchcraft and Black Magic*. New York, Grand River Books.

Trevor-Roper HR (1970) *The European Witch-craze of the Sixteenth and Seventeenth Centuries*. New York, Harper & Row.

Veith I (1965) *Hysteria: The History of a Disease*. Chicago, University of Chicago Press.

3 Mad, Bad or Just Different

A. BROWNBILL

INTRODUCTION

In this chapter, consideration will be given to some of the different ways in which mental distress is viewed or thought about or explained. Human beings have a tendency to try to make sense of the world – to find explanations for why things are the way they are or why they happen the way that they do. To help do this, maps or models are used. For example, in order to better understand the country that we live in, maps are available showing where places are in relation to each other. The maps that are constructed are not true images of the country that we live in but are representations of it that aim to improve our understanding of, and to navigate our way around, the country.

Depending on individual needs, there are many different maps. If there was a need to go to a different town by car, a road map would probably be the most useful; however, if a boating holiday were intended, the road map would not be very helpful. In that case, a map of the waterways would be needed. Maps may not be either right or wrong, but they may be more or less useful for our purposes. Similarly, in trying to understand mental distress over the years, different models have been constructed. At various times, people with mental illness have been thought to be possessed by evil spirits, influenced by the moon (from where we get the word 'lunatic') or to be suffering from imbalances in 'bodily humours'. Like maps these models are not necessarily right or wrong. This does not preclude debate arising as to which map is a truer representation or which map is simply false, however. Just like maps, models are more or less useful depending on what the particular interest is or what is their intended use.

The many models used to attempt to explain mental distress have many different titles. Consideration will be given in this chapter to the biomedical model, the cognitive model, moral models, the impaired model, family model, psychodynamic model and the user view.

In considering these different models, an attempt shall be made to try to answer the following questions: 'What is the basic viewpoint of the model?', 'How does the model try to explain the causes of human mental distress?', 'How does the model view the person?' and 'How does it try to intervene so as to reduce or eliminate the

Caring for Adults with Mental Health Problems   Edited by I. Peate and S. Chelvanayagam
© 2006 John Wiley & Sons, Ltd

problem?' The chapter is structured using three scenarios to consider the different models and issues raised. The first scenario concerns a man, Michael, who has attempted suicide. This situation will be used to consider the biomedical model, the psychodynamic model and the cognitive model. The second scenario concerns a young university student, Simon, who believes that he is being experimented upon. This situation will be used to consider the biomedical model in greater depth, the psychodynamic model and the impaired model. The third scenario is about a young woman, Angela, who was sexually abused as a child and has many difficulties in her adult life. This situation will be used to consider the moral view and the medical view. Finally, this chapter will consider how these and similar occurrences may be explained by the person who is experiencing them.

Consider the following case study about Michael.

Scenario One

Michael, a 33-year-old man, has been admitted to an acute admissions ward following a suicide attempt. He had parked his car on a country lane and attached a hose pipe to the exhaust in order to kill himself. Fortunately, he was discovered by a woman walking her dog and taken to hospital, from where, after being found to be physically stable, he was transferred to a psychiatric unit. Michael is the only son of George and Hilda. George is a very successful lawyer and a somewhat domineering man. He has always strongly encouraged Michael to do well in his education and career. Hilda gave up work when she was expecting Michael and has prided herself on providing a good home for George and Michael. Unfortunately, and unexpectedly, following a company reorganisation, Michael had been made redundant from his work in retail management six months previously. He had unsuccessfully struggled to find himself a similar position in management with other companies. Michael is married to Stephanie and they have two girls aged eight and five. Michael's suicide attempt came as a complete surprise to Stephanie, who believed that her husband was doing well in his job-seeking and he was expressing confidence that he would soon gain a good position.

THE BIOMEDICAL MODEL

In the biomedical model, human mental distress is seen as an illness or disease. In a similar way that we may suffer from physical illnesses which may cause pain or loss of function or unusual things happening to our bodies, mental illnesses can cause mental pain, loss of our ability to function normally and unusual things happening to our thoughts and moods. The sufferer is labelled as a 'patient', that is a person who is receiving medical care and the illness that they are suffering from is determined by doctors who look for signs and symptoms. The signs and symptoms of mental illness tend to be disturbances of moods, thought patterns and behaviours. Unlike with physical illness, there tend not to be definitive biochemical tests that help diagnose mental illness. Michael's attempt at suicide would be a behaviour that could lead to a diagnosis of depression. The admitting doctor would also be looking for other changes in behaviour, such as neglect of personal care, difficulty in sleeping, loss of appetite and loss of interest in previously enjoyed activities. Physically, the patient may feel weak and tired. His mood would be low and he would view the future with little optimism.

The biomedical model often uses knowledge from biological sciences to explain how mental illnesses come about. It will tend to look for the causes in anatomy, physiology, biochemistry and genetics. It considers that illness may be caused by involuntary physical changes such as chemical imbalances (Ogden 2000). In the case of depression, the biochemical imbalance is thought to occur in the synaptic clefts of nerves in the brain. The synaptic cleft is the space between one nerve and the next. It has been noted that in depressed people the concentration of some neurotransmitters is reduced in the synaptic cleft. Antidepressants act to increase the concentration of neurotransmitters in the synaptic cleft (Dinan 1997). In the biomedical model, the individual tends to be seen as a victim of their illness and is not responsible for it. The treatment would tend to be drug therapy in order to correct the biochemical imbalance. Meanwhile, nursing care would be offered to help support the patient to cope with their daily activities and to protect them from harm. The distinction between these two roles has been expressed by a psychiatrist once overheard to comment, 'My medication will cure the patient. Your job as nurses is to keep the patient alive long enough for my medication to work.' There will be more explanations of the medical view later on in this chapter.

THE PSYCHODYNAMIC MODEL

'Psychodynamics' is defined in the *Collins English Dictionary* (1991) as 'the study of interacting motives and emotions'. It is quite difficult to define more clearly than this and probably has different meanings for different people. However, we can say that the word derives from the word 'psyche' – the human mind or soul, and the word 'dynamics', which relates to forces and activity. So psychodynamics would consider how a person's mind would relate to parts of itself as well as other minds and other objects. It may seem a bit confusing to talk about how the mind relates to other parts of the same mind, but perhaps it can be explained by saying that we tend to experience ourselves as not being a single entity but as being made up of different parts. For example, we might happen to see a large chocolate cake that looks particularly delicious. Part of us may say, 'I want that cake and I want it now.' Another voice in our heads may say, 'I shouldn't have chocolate cake, because I am being greedy and it is fattening.' While a third voice could express the opinion that it would be all right to have a small piece of chocolate cake after having eaten all one's vegetables. These different voices or parts of the same mind would argue with each other in an internal dynamic.

Jacobs (2004) considers that the word 'psychodynamic' encompasses different psychoanalytic views and links psychotherapy and counselling with psychoanalysis. According to Spinelli (1994), two of the basic assumptions underlying psychoanalytic thought are the concept of unconscious mental processes and the idea that current behaviour, personality and attitudes stem from past childhood experiences.

If we consider Michael's situation from a psychodynamic viewpoint, we may believe that the causes of his suicide attempt lie in his childhood relationships with his parents. The role model for manhood provided by his father was one of being a strong head of the family, wage earner and professionally successful. His mother gave up work in order to concentrate on being a good wife and mother. Michael may have incorporated and internalised this set of values into his own belief system and his own attempts at building a family and, when faced with not being as successful as his father, could not cope with the difference between what he felt he should be and what he was. Because he may have been afraid or unable to express anger towards his father, owing to his father being domineering, these feelings of anger would have been repressed. As an adult, when he was made redundant by his employers, who could be seen as representative of a dominant father, his feelings of anger towards his father and his employers would resurface. However, being afraid of expressing these outwardly, he would have turned the aggression against himself in a suicide attempt.

Similarly, his father may have been a role model for strength and competence. By feeling that he too should be competent, Michael would have been unwilling to confide his worries to his wife thereby cutting himself off from a source of support and resulting in his wife not realising that he was having problems. The therapeutic methods that would be utilised to help Michael would be the talking therapies. Through counselling and psychotherapy, Michael would be able to develop awareness of how his past experiences were affecting his current situation, and thus he would be empowered to make changes. If we lack understanding of the unconscious forces that determine our emotions and behaviour, we have little control over them. When we have insight into our mental dynamics, we have more choice about our repertoire of responses.

Having mentioned how Michael may have used the ego defence mechanism of repressing his anger for fear of the consequences, it may be useful to explain ego defence mechanisms in a bit more detail. According to Dilts (2001), 'Ego defenses are the means by which the ego protects itself from anxiety.' There are quite a few of these defence mechanisms, which were originally considered by Freud's daughter, Anna. 'Repression' occurs when we are faced with a conflict or thought that would make us unacceptably anxious; so it is pushed into the unconscious mind. This act of repression is also unconscious. There may be situations where, when faced with a difficulty, we may choose to put it out of our minds until later on when we feel that we have time to deal with it, but this mechanism is known as 'suppression'. With repression, not only do we forget but we forget that we have forgotten.

Other familiar ego defences may be 'displacement' and 'projection'. An example of displacement might be if we were the victim of road rage and, being unable to express our feelings at the time, we pick a fight with a member of our family when we get home. The thought of the consequences of expressing our feelings to the driver of the other car may make us far too anxious; so the feelings are 'displaced' onto someone we feel less anxious about being angry with. This is commonly known as 'kicking the cat'. Projection occurs when we are faced with the fact that we have a characteristic that is intolerable for us to admit to so we deny the presence of it in ourselves and 'project' it onto someone or something outside of ourselves. For example, a person who is unable to come to terms with their own feelings of anger and aggression may deny that they have those qualities themselves but clearly see that another group of people do have those qualities. They may even go further and attack that group in order to eliminate aggression and bring about a more peaceful world. This is commonly known as 'hypocrisy'. There are many more ego defence mechanisms, which it would be useful to become familiar with if you have a particular interest in the psychodynamic model.

THE COGNITIVE VIEW

According to Trower *et al.* (1988) 'the central tenet of the cognitive behavioural approach can be summed up in the now famous words of the philosopher Epictetus in the first century AD. "Men are disturbed not by things but by the views which they take of them." ' This means that it is not the events that happen to us which cause distress but the interpretation or the meanings that we attach to those events. Different people experiencing the same situation will respond to it differently according to how they see the situation. So, with regard to Michael outlined above, it may have been the case that quite a few people were made redundant at the same time but only Michael responded with a suicide attempt. It is not the redundancy that caused the suicidal behaviour but Michael's thoughts and beliefs about being made redundant and the consequences of this for him and his family which led him to believe that his death would be the best outcome for everyone. Michael's beliefs may have been irrational. He may have thought that redundancy meant that he was a useless person, a failure as a man, that he would never be able to get another job and that he would not be able to be a good husband to his wife or a good father to his children. He may have thought that with less money coming in he would be unable to meet the bills and that the mortgage company would repossess his house, making his family homeless.

An important part of the cognitive behavioural approach is the ABC model. A = activating event, B = beliefs, C = consequences (Willson & Branch 2006). If we apply this model to Michael's situation, A would be the redundancy and the subsequent difficulty in gaining employment. The B would be those negative beliefs and assumptions about how he was a failure as a husband and father and the C would be the overwhelming feelings of sadness (emotional consequences) and his subsequent attempt to kill himself (behavioural consequences). A cognitive therapist would try to help the client by showing how their beliefs led to the consequences, assisting him to challenge the evidence for holding those beliefs and helping the client to develop more realistic, evidence-based beliefs (Trower *et al.* 1988).

Scenario Two

Simon is a 22-year-old university student of biological sciences who has been admitted to hospital after being arrested by the police for causing a disturbance in a shopping centre. It appears that he was shouting at people and accusing them of following him. On arrest, he was difficult to understand but seemed to be under the impression that he was being experimented upon. He was extremely agitated, dishevelled in appearance and kept accusing the police of 'being in league with "them" '. On admission to an acute mental health admission ward, he explained that a group of scientists were experimenting on him by putting drugs in his tea and monitoring him for the effects. He had heard these people discussing him from the next room to his. Up until a few weeks earlier, Simon had been a very conscientious student, obtaining good grades in his exams and was predicted to get a first- or upper-second-class honours degree. He was a popular person amongst his fellow students and had had a steady girlfriend up until three months ago when she left him for someone else. Following this, Simon seemed to lose interest in his studies, neglected his personal hygiene and started to avoid his friends. It had been suggested that Simon may have taken some marijuana or a hallucinogenic drug, but his friends insist that Simon would never take illegal substances as he has always been very intolerant of drug abuse.

THE BIOMEDICAL MODEL

Following a psychiatric assessment, Simon would probably be diagnosed with schizophrenia, a schizophreniform disorder or a schizoaffective disorder, depending on the duration of the illness, the presence or absence of a decline in functioning and the presence or absence of prominent mood symptoms. According to the American Psychiatric Association's *Diagnostic and Statistical Manual of Mental Disorders IV* (American Psychiatric Association 2000), the illness of schizophrenia would be characterised by prominent active symptoms of delusions, hallucinations and thought disorder and negative symptoms of emotional flattening and lack of volition or will. Simon's behaviour could also have resulted from taking some illegal drugs, but his friends insist that that would not be the case. As mentioned earlier, the biomedical model would seek to explain schizophrenia by reference to biochemistry or brain disorder or trauma.

Genetics would also be an important part of the biomedical explanation in that if it could be demonstrated that persons suffering from schizophrenia had inherited a 'schizophrenic gene' the case for schizophrenia being an illness would be given more support. In order to identify the significance of genetic inheritance, researchers often use identical twins and fraternal twins. Identical twins inherit exactly the same genes from both their parents. So if an identical twin suffered from schizophrenia and the cause of schizophrenia was genetic we would expect the other twin to suffer from schizophrenia as well. Of course, it could be argued that twins are usually brought up in the same household under very similar conditions, and so if they both have schizophrenia it could be due to the fact that they had similar upbringings. This is the basic argument of the 'nature versus nurture' debate. Are we a result of our genetic inheritance or are we a result of our upbringing? The most likely answer is that we are a product of at least both influences, but the relative importance of each is often debated. What is looked for, to demonstrate the impact of inheritance, is known as the 'concordance rate'. If schizophrenia has a genetic cause, we would expect the chances of developing schizophrenia to be greater according to the percentage of genes that we have in common with someone who has schizophrenia. The closer we are genetically to someone with the illness, the more likely we are to have the same illness. Research has shown (McGue *et al.* 1985, cited in Thomas 1997) that the concordance rate for identical twins is 44.3%, whereas for non-identical twins it is 12.08%. This would suggest that there is a strong genetic component to the development of schizophrenia. However, if it were solely of genetic causation, the concordance rate for identical twins would be much higher than 44.3%. The biomedical model would argue that one can inherit a predisposition to develop the illness and that other environmental factors may then be of some influence.

Another science that would support the biomedical model would be biochemistry. Biochemically, schizophrenia is considered to be a result of problems with the dopamine receptors. Dopamine is one of a group of substances that are involved with the transmission of impulses from one nerve to another. It has been found that the drugs which are most effective in reducing the symptoms of schizophrenia tend to block the dopamine receptors at the ends of the nerves (Gelder *et al.* 1996). However, Gelder *et al.* point out that evidence for the assumption that dopamine neurotransmission is faulty in individuals with schizophrenia is quite weak. There seems to be a lot of evidence to support the thesis that schizophrenia is a medical illness related to genetics and biochemistry. However, it is also apparent that there are other influences.

For a fuller explanation of the dopamine hypothesis as well as other biological explanations of mental disorders see Dinan (1997). If the biomedical view of schizophrenia is used, the treatment of choice would be to readjust the individual's faulty biochemistry with a pharmacological intervention. The patient would be prescribed antipsychotic medication.

The biomedical model would see a schizophrenic's behaviour and conversation as being symptomatic of the illness and not necessarily as having any valid meaning in themselves. There is still some controversy regarding whether or not psychotic illnesses such as schizophrenia can be successfully treated with talking therapies. Those who strictly follow the biomedical view would say that, as it is a biochemical disorder, only interventions that alter biochemistry would work. However, there is a developing body of knowledge that supports the view that counselling, cognitive behavioural therapy and other talking therapies have a part to play. Bradshaw and Roseborough (2004) note, 'There was a statistically significant reduction in the negative impact of illness on sense of self. Findings support the effectiveness of cognitive-behavioural interventions in schizophrenia.' Of course, it could be argued that the talking therapies do not provide a cure but help the patient to manage their lives with the illness. On the other hand, it could also be argued that being on antipsychotic medication for many years, if not for life, does not constitute a cure either but is another way to help people manage an 'incurable' illness.

THE FAMILY OR SYSTEMIC MODEL

Student nurses in the 1970s were advised not to encourage schizophrenic symptoms by responding to the patient's delusions but, instead, to gently distract. A young woman was admitted to an acute mental health admission ward. According to her parents, she had been behaving very strangely and had not been herself lately. The young woman indeed acted strangely and insisted that her name was Taylor in spite of her parent's insistence that it was not. Regardless of the advice given about not colluding with the patient's symptoms, this matter was explored with the patient. She also liked to be referred to by the rather old-fashioned term of a 'maiden'. It did not take long for the maiden of the Taylor family to talk about herself as a 'Taylor maiden', which gradually developed into the description that she was 'Tailor-made'. Rather than being a symptom of a delusional mind, this young woman's strange communication turned out to be a clear message about the relationship that she felt she had with her parents. This leads us to consider the family, or systemic, model.

According to L'Abate and McHenry (1983), the development of communication theory in marital and family therapy can be traced to the research done by Gregory Bateson in 1956. It was this research that led to the concept of the 'double bind' and the role of incongruent messages in the causation of schizophrenia. The 'double bind' is a communication in which two conflicting messages are given. It is impossible to respond to both messages at the same time because they are contradictory. Whatever a person does is wrong. An example might be where a child is given strong verbal messages about being loved but the behaviour of the parents is very harsh or judgemental and not experienced as loving. Bateson would argue that a history of such confusing messages is damaging and, if prolonged and intense, is schizophrenogenic or able to cause schizophrenia. The double bind is seen as a situation in which schizophrenia may be seen as a way of adapting to an insane situation rather than as an illness. This is well explained by Dallos and Draper (2005).

This family model, where the interactions of the family members are seen to be a cause, is fundamentally different from the biomedical model and the impaired model, in that the focus is shifted away from the individual. In the biomedical model, the individual is seen to have an illness. In the impaired model, it is the individual who is seen to be damaged in some way. In the family model, the individual is the 'index patient' who points to the fact that the whole family is somehow disturbed and disturbing. It has been suggested that the index patient – the one with the symptoms, who causes the family to seek help – may actually be the sanest of all and has developed symptoms as a result of not being able to cope with living in a crazy family. Treatment, according to this view, would be aimed at helping the whole family to change their ways of relating so that the index patient can stop responding with symptoms.

In his book *Toxic Psychiatry*, Peter Breggin (1991) gives a good example of how this worked with a young boy called Andy, who was considered to be a hyperactive child. Breggin's work with Andy's parents provided an alternative to the medical prescription of Ritalin as a treatment for attention deficit disorder. So, to consider Simon in the scenario above, biomedically he could be considered to have inherited faulty genes resulting in faulty biochemistry and requiring medication to correct the faults. Alternatively, the family's communication patterns that Simon experienced as a child could be seen to have created the personality that would respond to a stressful event with a schizophrenic episode. You may recall that Simon had recently broken up with his girlfriend. A useful metaphor is to think about triggers and bullets. The stress itself would not have directly caused the schizophrenic breakdown but may have been the trigger. The bullets which resulted in this particular response were loaded in childhood as a result of the disordered and confusing communications that Simon may have had with his parents. One of the results of this way of thinking was that families started to feel blamed for the mental illness of individuals within the family. Keen (1999) discusses this point in his paper 'Schizophrenia: orthodoxy and heresies' in which he states, 'It would make no more sense to blame families for their parenting style than it would to blame God.' Blame is inappropriate as in order to blame there should be evidence of intent. Breggin (1991) suggests that the sense of blame can provoke individuals, support groups and mental health charities to expend much effort in trying to prove that schizophrenia is a medical illness. If this could be demonstrated beyond doubt, relatives of people with schizophrenia would be able to absolve themselves of any blame associated with the possibility that they had, in some way, helped to bring about the disordered thinking through disordered communications.

THE IMPAIRED MODEL

If human difference is considered from the viewpoint that some people are impaired, or damaged, or handicapped in some way, medical diagnosis of illness becomes more irrelevant. The patient is seen as being reduced or constricted or held back in some way with regard to the capabilities that are considered normal and as a result they need to be cared for. Medical treatment for diagnosed illnesses takes more of a back seat; instead, it is accepted that the person will not be able to function normally as a result of their impairment. Attempts to make people better are considered futile and the aim becomes one of trying to enable the damaged individuals to live their lives as fully as possible within the limits of their impairment. This way of looking at people was quite common in the old psychiatric hospitals. Patients would be admitted to acute mental health admission wards, where they would receive treatment for their illness. If, after a period of time, however, it was believed that treatment was not helping in curing the illness or reducing the symptoms sufficiently so that the patient could return to their former lives, they were transferred to one of the 'back wards' where the emphasis was shifted from treatment of an illness to the care of an individual who would need long-term support. Medical treatment, usually in the form of medication, was continued in order to control symptoms as much as possible, but the emphasis of the care was to provide everything that the patient needed in order to function. It was not anticipated that the patient would ever leave the hospital and so the responsibility for meeting all of their daily needs fell to the hospital staff. Patients were provided with food, warmth, occupation, clothing, religious services, entertainment, exercise and cigarettes. What they were not provided with was the freedom to make choices about their life. To have some self-determination, some sense of control over one's life, could be seen as an essential component of our sense of identity. Interestingly, patients were not called patients any more. They tended to be collectively termed 'the boys'; so student nurses would be instructed to 'take the boys down to the workshop' or 'take the boys for a walk'. The use of the word 'boys' seemed appropriate with regard to them having had the adult's freedom to choose removed and thereby being rendered more childlike.

If this scenario had happened about 40 years ago and it was felt that Simon was unable to manage independently in the community due to his having schizophrenia, he could easily have been considered to be impaired and thus in need of institutional care for many years. The author recalls being taught in the 1970s that 'schizophrenia is an incurable disease where there will be a gradual but inevitable deterioration of the personality and the poor sufferer is better off in hospital where he can be looked after for the rest of his life'. Erving Goffman (1961) provides an excellent description of these institutions in his book *Asylums*.

THE MORAL MODEL

The question of whether some behaviours result from mental illness or moral weakness often arises. Are people with an addiction to alcohol suffering from an illness resulting from genetic inheritance, faulty metabolism or missing biochemicals or do they wilfully choose to adopt a behaviour that offends against a moral standard of sobriety? Are children who play truant from school or behave in an uncontrolled way naughty and deserving of punishment or do they suffer from attention deficit disorder, hyperactivity disorder or school phobia and need to be treated for their illness?

The following scenario will be used to explore the 'mad or bad?' debate.

Scenario Three

Angela is 25 years old. Following the death of her mother from cancer when Angela was 11 years old, her father sexually abused her, initially demanding that she masturbate him and later forcing her to have full sexual intercourse. She ran away from home at 14 and became involved with a man who introduced her to marijuana and heroin. Since then, she has been a fairly regular user of illegal drugs and resorts to prostitution and shoplifting in order to finance her habit. Since the age of 14, she has had repeated admissions to Accident and Emergency departments for treatment of drug overdoses and self-inflicted lacerations to her arms and wrists. She is well known by the staff in A & E and tends not to be treated with much compassion. She is also well known to the psychiatric services of her local hospital where she has been admitted on many occasions but discharges herself within a few days. The staff describe her as being very manipulative, attention-seeking and impossible to work with. Originally, she was diagnosed as having depression but has now been given the diagnosis of antisocial personality disorder.

THE MORAL VIEW VERSUS THE BIOMEDICAL VIEW

This scenario raises the question: 'Mad or bad?' The fact that Angela has been diagnosed with an illness – antisocial personality disorder – would suggest that she has a disease or illness. The fact that she gets admitted to hospitals would support this. Hospitals are places where ill people are treated for their illnesses in order to restore them to health. However, much of Angela's behaviour could be considered as bad. Her use of illegal drugs, her prostitution and her shoplifting could invite legal action. Of course, one could always say that bad people can become ill as well as ill people can do bad things, but this does not always clarify the situation and the question of labelling people as ill or bad remains. The issue tends to be one of asking how society should work with such people who go against what is expected of members of society. If we consider that they behave in antisocial ways because they are ill, it would be natural to assume that they should receive treatment for their illness. It would be inhumane to punish someone for having an illness. However, if it were felt that their behaviour was the result of a deliberate breach of the law, and not due to illness, such people should be punished according to the law.

An extreme example may help to illuminate the issue. Ian Brady and Myra Hindley, the Moors Murderers, were tried for murder in 1966 and, being found guilty, were both sentenced to life imprisonment. In 1985, Ian Brady was transferred to a high-security hospital. However, Myra Hindley stayed in prison until she died following a chest infection at the age of 60 in 2002. The judge who sentenced Hindley was reported as saying, 'Though I believe Brady is wicked beyond belief without hope of redemption (short of a miracle), I cannot feel the same is necessarily true of Hindley once she is removed from his influence' (Fenton Atkinson 2006). In this case, both of the perpetrators of the crime were considered to be bad and were imprisoned. However, later on, Ian Brady was thought to be ill and so was transferred to hospital for treatment. Myra Hindley, who the judge had said that he did not believe was wicked beyond redemption, stayed in prison until the end of her life. There can be much discussion about why these two people who committed the same crimes were eventually treated differently by society – one being seen as bad and the other as mentally ill – and much of the discussion can be and has been centred around the idea that Myra Hindley was considered more bad because society would not expect a *woman* to behave in such a way, whereas we are more accustomed to expect men to behave violently. However, it does indicate that sometimes we have difficulty in deciding whether a model of mental illness or unacceptable behaviour is best for helping us to decide how to deal with people.

The use of the term 'attention-seeking' in the description of Angela also presents an interesting issue. The requirement for attention is probably a fundamental human need. However, to seek attention is considered bad and the term 'attention-seeking' when used in the context of people with mental health problems is usually pejorative or judgemental. A person who is attention-seeking would be seen as acting in an inappropriate way and would probably be ignored in order to try to reduce the attention-seeking behaviour. Interestingly, if a patient were to ask for a drink because they were thirsty they would not be denied the drink on the grounds that they were 'fluid-seeking'. Of course, it may depend on how the patient seeks fluid or attention. There are some ways of meeting our needs that are considered acceptable and some that are not. It is considered inappropriate to seek attention by taking overdoses of drugs or by cutting oneself or by acting in a way that could be considered crazy. It is socially acceptable to seek attention in other ways, such as by becoming a celebrity. It could be seen as paradoxical that being given a diagnosis of mental illness does not necessarily permit someone to behave in a crazy way. People who do self-harm would often claim that they are not doing it in order to seek attention but are doing it because they find that it relieves their mental distress. However, health professionals often have difficulty in working with people who seem to deliberately harm themselves.

Many people would consider that paedophiles are immoral people who should be punished for their behaviour. There might be many possible reasons why someone may prefer to have sex with prepubescent children. Perhaps they have an illness caused by a genetic abnormality. This could have affected their biochemistry in such a way that they are only sexually aroused by children. Perhaps they suffered some brain trauma, at birth, which means that parts of the brain do not function, thereby affecting their development to adulthood. Perhaps they were abused themselves in childhood or maybe their childhood relationships with adults were so traumatic that they feel unable to relate comfortably to adults. This could have so stunted the development of the paedophile (arrested development) that they might be considered like children themselves and, if so, less responsible for their behaviour. In this case, punishment would be inappropriate. As a society, we may choose to protect children by restricting the freedom of the paedophile but that does not have to be seen as a punishment. If, on the other hand, a paedophile is a person who has the capacity to meet his or her needs in ways that are legally sanctioned but deliberately chooses to break the law, we may consider that such a person is immoral and that punishment is appropriate.

To confuse the issues a bit further, it may be useful to point out that our thoughts on whether aberrant behaviour is due to illness or moral transgressions are not consistent across time and place. A couple of examples may help to clarify this point. Society's views on homosexuality have changed over the years. In AD 1290, there was the first mention in English common law of a punishment for homosexuality. In 1533, an Act was passed in England that made buggery punishable by hanging. In 1961, Illinois was the first state in the US to decriminalise homosexuality. In 1967, the Sexual Offences Act came into force in England and Wales and decriminalised homosexual acts between two men over 21 years of age and in private. In 2000, the British Government lifted the ban on homosexuals serving in the armed forces (The Knitting Circle 2006).

In 1973, the American Psychiatric Association removed homosexuality from its diagnostic category of mental illnesses. Here we can see that homosexuality had been considered to be a moral issue and that people who carried out homosexual acts could be punished by law. Later on, views changed and it was considered to be an illness so that the homosexual was a person who needed treatment rather than punishment. More recently, attitudes have been changing again so that homosexuality is not considered to be a crime or an illness but is an alternative way of being, which should be just as acceptable as heterosexuality. Not mad or bad. Just different.

A similar transition can also be seen in the case of shell shock. According to Marlowe (2000), prior to 1915 soldiers in battle who demonstrated fear and unwillingness to fight the enemy would have been seen as cowards or malingerers and would have been treated either punitively or with contempt. Quite a few soldiers were shot for cowardice. From 1915 onwards, the First World War was a time when what had previously been seen as cowardice, punishable by death, was now being seen as an illness. There was considerable debate about whether it was a physical illness resulting from nerves being damaged by such close proximity to explosions or whether it was a psychological disorder resulting from the mind's difficulty in coping with very real danger and fear.

More recently, such a response may be given the diagnosis of post-traumatic stress disorder (PTSD). However, there is a developing view that to medicalise the issue is not helpful. Service personnel suffering from exposure to such difficult situations are not seen as bad (cowards) or ill (having PTSD) but rather as normal people reacting appropriately to very abnormal situations. As in the changes in attitude to homosexuality, it can be seen that in this case there has been a transition from 'bad' to 'mad' to 'a different sort of normal'.

There are similar movements in how other psychiatric illnesses are viewed. From a psychiatric viewpoint, hearing voices is one of the symptoms of schizophrenia and considered to be a symptom that should be either removed or, at least, diminished in intensity. There is a humorous quote that if you talk to God it is called prayer but if God talks to you it is called schizophrenia (Szasz 1973). In 1988, an organisation called the Hearing Voices Network was started in Manchester (for details see References section at the end of this chapter). Their website makes the following comment: 'Hearing voices has been regarded by psychiatry as "auditory hallucinations" and, in many cases, a symptom of schizophrenia. However, not everyone who hears voices has a diagnosis of schizophrenia.' One of the aims of the organisation is to offer alternative approaches to how hearing voices is viewed so that it is not necessarily seen as an illness. This could be seen as another example of the movement from perceiving strange experiences or behaviour as illness to viewing them as just different – but it is all right to be different. Rachel Studley, who has a diagnosis of schizoaffective disorder, has written the following on the 'MadNOTBad' website:

> I also am a person. I might well be sitting next to you in your local pub chatting about the charms of the latest draft ale. I spend the odd Saturday night in front of the TV (well, hiding behind a rather large cushion) with a good scary movie and some tasty ice cream. I live (thankfully). I breathe. I cry. I laugh (just don't ask me to recite a joke 'cause I can't). I also have really suspect taste in hair accessories and have a strong fondness for sparkly things. I am one person among millions, and I'm no more mad, bad or dangerous to know than you are. (Studley 2006)

THE USER VIEW

Rachel Studley's writing about herself introduces the user view. Many people have felt that traditional approaches to mental health care have been more damaging than helpful. For many years, people who have suffered from the treatments as much as from the illness have spoken about their distress. It can be imagined that somebody with mental illness who was about to be burned at the stake for being possessed by demons may have felt that the cure was worse than the condition being treated; however, it is only in the last 30 years or so that the 'user movement' has really started to have an impact on mental health services. To call it a movement is probably a bit of a misnomer in that it is actually a lot of movements. What may have initially started as people complaining about the treatment they had received has grown so that, today, users and ex-users of psychiatric services are involved in a whole range of activities from lobbying decision-makers in Government and educating health care professionals to providing alternatives to statutory care. Users sit on Trust-management committees, support patients in hospitals and have a voice in the development of services.

Some will say that even though it is now broadly acknowledged that users have a voice that voice is not often listened to. The author recalls attending a conference in the 1980s at which about 20 professionals spent the day talking about the contributions that they were making to developing community care initiatives. It was a very pleasant conference with lots of discussion about all the good things that we were doing. At the end of the day, during the evaluation session, the one psychiatric patient who had attended the conference made the following remark. 'It is all a load of rubbish really. You have all got lots of ideas. Some of your ideas are good ideas and some of them are bad ideas, but that is not the point. The point is that they are always your ideas. The professionals' ideas. It is only when you allow us, the users, to have our ideas that things will improve. We may have good ideas or we may have bad ideas but they will be our ideas.' Fifteen years later, Campbell (1998) makes the following point, 'In twenty years' time it may well appear that the greatest contribution of the user movement in the last decade has not been to criticise the psychiatric approach to distress but to assert and demonstrate the capacities and competencies of people with a diagnosis of mental illness.'

These are just a few of the models or views that can be useful in helping us to understand the nature of mental distress. There are many other ways in which people can make sense of the myriad variations in human experiences. Some may use a social model in which it is assumed that mental illness results from a society that allows things like poverty, unemployment and discrimination to exist. Some may believe that there is no such thing as mental illness and that psychiatry is another form of social control which enables us to deal with people considered unacceptably different. Many people believe that the difficult times which they may have suffered in their lives have been an essential part of their learning and development and that, rather than wishing it had never occurred, they are grateful for the personal growth that has resulted. Professionals in the mental health field have lots of different views about what is mental illness, what causes mental illness and what is the best way of treating, dealing with and managing mental illness. Many professionals would see that part of their role is to help the patient or client to see the world from the professional's perspective and thereby help them return to reality. On the other hand, the users of psychiatric services, or 'survivors' as some would call themselves, may consider that the mental health professionals should expend more effort on trying to see the world from the client's point of view.

In conclusion, this has been a brief introduction to how human mental distress has been, and may be, perceived and explained. The advantages and disadvantages of the different models have been considered and the way in which the views of the person who is mentally distressed have been increasingly valued has been noted.

REFERENCES

American Psychiatric Association (2000) *Diagnostic and Statistical Manual of Mental Disorders – IV* (4th edn.). Washington, American Psychiatric Association.

Bradshaw W, Roseborough D (2004) Evaluating the effectiveness of cognitive-behavioral treatment of residual symptoms and impairment in schizophrenia. *Research on Social Work Practice* **14**(2): 112–120.

Breggin P (1991) *Toxic Psychiatry*. New York, HarperCollins.

Campbell P (1998) Listening to clients. In *Ethical Strife* (P Barker, B Davidson, eds). London, Arnold.

Dallos R, Draper R (2005) *An Introduction to Family Therapy: Systemic Theory and Practice* (2nd edn.). London, Open University Press.

Dilts SL (2001) *Models of the Mind: A framework for Biopsychosocial Psychiatry*. Philadelphia PA, Brunner-Routledge.

Dinan T (1997) *Understanding the Biology of Mental Disorders*. London, Science Press.

Fenton Atkinson J (2006) Letter to the Home Secretary, 8 May 1966, http://www.hmcourts-service.gov.uk/judgmentsfiles/j59/hindleym.htm, accessed 20 July 2006.

Gelder M, Gath D, Mayou R, Cowen P (eds) (1996) *Oxford Textbook of Psychiatry* (3rd. edn.). Oxford, Oxford University Press.

Goffman E (1961) *Asylums*. New York, Anchor Books.

Hearing Voices Network Enquiries and Information: 0845 122 8641; email: info@hearing-voices.org; website: www.hearing-voices.org.

Jacobs M (2004) *Psychodynamic Counselling in Action* (3rd edn.). London, SAGE.

Keen T (1999) Schizophrenia: orthodoxy and heresies: a review of alternative possibilities. *Journal of Psychiatric and Mental Health Nursing* **6**(6): 415–424.

Knitting Circle, The (2006) The Knitting Circle: history, http://myweb.lsbu.ac.uk/~stafflag/timetable, accessed 20 July 2006.

L'Abate L, McHenry S (1983) *Handbook of Marital Interventions*. New York, Grune & Stratton.

Marlowe DH (2000) Psychological and psychosocial consequences of combat and deployment with special emphasis on the Gulf War, http://www.gulflink.osd.mil/library/randrep/marlowe_paper/mr1018_11_ch5.html, accessed 22 July 2006.

Ogden J (2000) *Health Psychology* (2nd edn.). Buckingham: Open University Press.

Spinelli E (1994) *Demystifying Therapy*. London, Constable.

Szasz T (1973) *The Second Sin*. Garden City, NY, Doubleday.

Studley R (2006) Not mad, not bad and not all that dangerous to know, http://www.madnotbad.co.uk/views/v8_notmad.htm, accessed 22 July 2006.

Thomas P (1997) *The Dialectics of Schizophrenia*. London, Free Association Books.

Trower P, Casey A, Dryden W (1988) *Cognitive Behavioural Counselling in Action*. London, SAGE.

Willson R, Branch R (2006) *Cognitive Behavioural Therapy for Dummies*. Chichester, John Wiley & Sons.

4 Partnership Working in Mental Health Care

P. ILLINGWORTH

INTRODUCTION

Traditionally, welfare provision in the UK has been predominantly paternalistic, with interventions being undertaken on service users by professionals, with the latter seen very much as 'the experts'. Consequently, professionals have more often occupied positions of authority with service users deferring to their specialist knowledge and expertise. The term 'doctor knows best' is an example of this, implying that their intensive education enables them to identify and respond to problems with little or no input from the person actually experiencing the problem.

The different perspectives of service users and professionals are demonstrated in Table 4.1, demonstrating the professional–paternalistic approach, as opposed to the service user–civil liberty approach.

For many people with a mental illness, they may find their daily existence to be a struggle; they may also feel oppressed, disempowered and can often lack self-determination. Service users and many people involved in mental health care provision see the need for working and training together as a means not only of improving mental health care but also of empowering service users (Campbell 1997; Lindow 1991). This 'working together' has often been called:

- collaborative working
- collaborative care
- multidisciplinary team
- multi-agency working
- interprofessional working
- interagency working.

The term 'partnership working' is used because mental health care is seen more as a joint venture. When discussing this area of mental health work, some of the key groups are often omitted or given unequal status; partnership working allows for these groups to be included. Even though there is a wide acceptance that partnership

Caring for Adults with Mental Health Problems   Edited by I. Peate and S. Chelvanayagam
© 2006 John Wiley–Sons, Ltd

Table 4.1 Paternalism vs. Civil Liberty
(adapted from Lindow 1996)

Paternalism	Civil Liberty
Charity	Justice
Experts know best	Choice
Dependence	Independence

working is not only needed but also more effective than single-agency working (Audit Commission 1998), it does not always happen in practice. This chapter is, therefore, written with those groups who are often omitted or given unequal status (service users, carers and non-professional groups) as being deemed to be central to the activity. For all groups involved in mental health care, the common agenda is their wish to help, but there are factors that can either help or hinder this.

If help could be obtained from one single group, many of the problems resulting in service failure would cease. However, mental health service users often have many different issues that may need interventions, and one group cannot provide all of the help required. If the mental health needs of service users are to be provided effectively, the different groups need to be aware of each other and have some understanding of the service user's different needs, as well as the different beliefs and roles of the professional groups.

In recent years, there have been many reports that have repeatedly stressed the importance of partnership working.

- *Partnership in Action (New Opportunities for Joint Working Between Health and Social Services)* (Department of Health 1998a)
- *The Report of the Inquiry into the Case and Treatment of Christopher Clunis* (Ritchie *et al.* 1994)
- *Panel Report from the Inquiry into the Care and Treatment of Richard King* (Capon 2005)
- *The Capable Practitioner* (Sainsbury Centre for Mental Health 2001)

The Government recognised the need to improve the way agencies worked together when caring for those people with a mental illness (Department of Health (Department of Health) 1998a) and saw the *National Service Frameworks* (NSFs) (Department of Health 1999a) as one way of enabling the delivery of better mental health provision. Additionally, a framework for lifelong learning was developed to help with the way agencies worked together (Department of Health 2001a). Despite this, there are examples of breakdowns in mental health care; some of these have resulted in headlines in national newspapers and resulted in public outcry. One such development to counter this was *The Capable Practitioner* (Sainsbury Centre for Mental Health 2001), which aims to cover the skills, knowledge and attitudes required by mental health practitioners to put into action the aspirations of the *National Service Framework for Mental Health* (Department of Health 1999a) and current policy. The publication combines the notion of the effective practitioner with that of the reflective practitioner. More recently, attempts to develop mental health services have taken these principles in mind, to some extent.

THE PARTNERSHIPS

There are several definitions of 'partnership working' that have been produced; for this chapter, the following working definition was developed by the author:

> Partnership working involves an understanding that there is equality of any relationship between all relevant parties who are working in a co-ordinated way, but who, at times, may have differing points of view on how to reach the agreed goal.

The National Institute for Mental Health in England (2003a) argues that, despite a wealth of barriers to partnership working identified in the literature, there is an unmistakable need for a clear pathway from the point of entry to the service through to the point of discharge. In reality, what this implies is that there is the need for a wide range of agencies working in partnership. It is important to know who the partners will be when working with people who have mental health care needs. Not knowing what different types of professionals there are available could prevent a service user getting the help they really need. Take a moment and write down the groups of people you might come into contact with as a mental health care worker. Check your list with the list in Table 4.2.

- Did you have more or fewer than those in Table 4.2?
- Did you have any that were not in Table 4.2?
- If you had more that were not in Table 4.2, why do you think that was so?

Table 4.2 Some of the mental health care partners

Non-professional	Health and Social Services	Others
Service users	Mental health nurses	Housing
Family carers	Occupational therapists	Education providers
Voluntary groups	Psychiatrists (doctors)	Leisure services
Charities	General practitioners	Police
User groups	Approved social workers	Criminal justice workers
	Clinical psychologists	Prison officers
	Graduate mental health workers	Youth offender teams
	Mental health hospitals	
	Independent/private health care providers	
	Drug and alcohol services	
	Child & Adolescent mental health services	

The lists in Table 4.2 are not exhaustive, as there will be many other national and local partners involved in mental health care. In your own working area, there are likely to be many other groups involved. The reason for this is the need to provide localised services which meet the specific needs of the local community and those that are not met by the statutory services. It will be important for you to identify as many as possible. In effect, involvement can be grouped into five main areas of health care partnership.

THE 5 P'S OF PARTNERSHIP

1. *People partnerships* – particularly service users and carers. By empowering and involving service users and carers their own power to challenge services will be enhanced and their needs met.
2. *Purchaser partnerships* – money is provided by central Government; this is distributed to organisations, who then, following assessments of local needs, allocate monies to organisations that then provide the actual service.
3. *Primary Care partnerships* – some Primary Care Trusts (PCTs) not only provide health care to a local population but also are currently critical to purchasing and the development of localised community-based mental health care.
4. *Provider partnerships* – local NHS mental health services and social services have come together in the common interest of service users. Health and social care providers use the money allocated to provide local specific services for the community they serve.
5. *Professional partnerships* – in an attempt to overcome traditional professional rivalries and to create interdisciplinary commitment to a common purpose. Professional groups have traditionally been set up to provide health and social services.

Any partnership working, at whatever level, involves people. It is this area, communication between people, professionals and agencies, that has often been seen as the major reason for mental health care failing (Capon 2005; Mental Health Foundation 1994; Ritchie *et al.* 1994).

Alongside the five P's, the independent/voluntary sector must be recognised and involved, especially where they reflect the needs of specific groups such as women, children and people from diverse ethnic backgrounds.

EFFECTIVE PARTNERSHIPS

COMMUNICATION

Numerous reports have been produced following inquiries into the failure of mental health services. What they all have in common is that communication breakdown is the main cause for the failure. The Ritchie Inquiry into the tragic death of Jonathan

Zito by Christopher Clunis, who had a long history of mental illness, identified communication, among other areas, as the cause of the fatal stabbing. As a result of this and other such findings, governments have produced publications such as *The Care Programme Approach* (Department of Health 1990) and, more recently, the *National Service Framework for Mental Health* (Department of Health 1999a). This latter document identifies clear aims of care and then stipulates standards that professionals have to achieve. This gives professionals clarity over their responsibilities and lines of accountability and stresses the need for open communication between all parties. As Onyett (2003) states, effective communication needs clear aims and shared values.

ATTITUDES

Positive attitudes are vital for effective partnership working. There is a need to reconsider the power of professionals over non-professionals and service users/carers. Involving service users will effectively mean a shift in power, according to Repper and Perkins (2003). However, some in the service user movement have argued that power is so entrenched in mental health working that working in partnership will never be fully achieved (Coleman & Harding 2004). Goss and Miller (1995) developed a 'ladder of participation' in relation to service user involvement (Table 4.3). Their ladder is made up of five levels ranging from no involvement to full participation.

Table 4.3 Ladder of service user involvement (Adapted from Goss & Miller 1995)

Level one	No involvement
Level two	Passive involvement (e.g. consultation with service users through third party)
Level three	Tokenism (e.g. consultation with service users through non-decision-making forums)
Level four	Collaboration (e.g. service users' views form the basis for decision-making)
Level five	Full partnership (service providers and service users work systematically, strategically and jointly at all stages of planning, delivery and management).

Only by working at level five will a positive attitude to working in partnership with service users and carers be achieved. Additionally, Payne (2000) suggests that partnership working can help to bring together skills, the sharing of information, the allocation of roles and thus the resulting assured responsibility/accountability. This would achieve a continuity of care and coordinate the planning and the delivery of resources by professionals for the benefit of service users. However, this could be viewed as seeing service users as being irrelevant to the partnership working.

BARRIERS TO PARTNERSHIP WORKING

Even though partnership working is seen as a positive approach to care delivery, there are a number of well-documented barriers. Hudson *et al.* (1997) identify five barriers to partnership working:

1. Structural – fragmentation of services between and across agencies/services.
2. Procedural – differences in planning visions and cycles, budgets, procedure, information systems and protocols.
3. Financial – different funding mechanisms and bases as well as flow of resources.
4. Professional – self-interests and autonomy of professional groups, interprofessional rivalry, threats to job security and roles.
5. Status and legitimacy – organisational self-interest and competition, difference in legitimacy between elected and appointed agencies.

Hudson *et al.* (1997) go on to suggest that to overcome these barriers, there are four broad principles for strengthening the strategic approach to partnership working:

1. Have a shared vision, specifying what is to be achieved in terms of service-user-centred goals and by clarifying the purpose of partnership working as a means of achieving such goals.
2. Clarify and agree upon roles and responsibilities (who does what).
3. Maintain appropriate incentives and rewards, promoting organisational behaviour consistent with the goals and responsibilities and gain organisation self-interest in the collective goals.
4. Ensure accountability for joint working. Have monitoring in place relating to the stated vision, and hold individuals and agencies accountable for the achievement of the vision/goals.

Currently, with respect to mental health provision, most, if not all, of the above have been implemented. Additionally, there are at least five other barriers that can obstruct effective partnership working:

1. To hold stereotypical views of each other prevents cooperation between partners.
2. Professions practising interdependently but autonomously may promote isolation between disciplines, as Spokes *et al.* (2002) found when researching violence on acute mental health admission wards.
3. A reliance on hierarchy restricts individuals, although to have a fully democratic partnership, where decisions are taken on a majority vote, is unlikely to be beneficial (Onyett 2003).
4. A complete rejection of hierarchy can be just as damaging, especially as the hierarchy usually continues to exist covertly, and power may be exercised subtly and unaccountably.
5. The people at the lower end of the hierarchy have great informal power to influence for good or bad the partnership's goals; to disregard their goals and aspirations is to put at risk the partnership.

Several other reasons have been consistently identified as factors reducing the ability for partnership working. Foremost among the reasons are:

- philosophical differences (Stevenson 1985; Strauss 1962)
- role confusion (Ross & Campbell 1992)
- conflicting power relations (Blane 1991; Galvin & McCarthy 1994)
- poor communication and language differences (Department of Health 1991; Pietroni 1992).

Having identified the barriers, it is important to note that there are examples of success in partnership working (Cook *et al.* 2001; Millar 2000).

MENTAL HEALTH SERVICES

Some of the different care settings within which mental health care is delivered are described briefly below. Caplan (1964) describes three functions of interventions that are often used to deliver health care: primary, secondary and tertiary. In simple terms, these relate as follows:

- primary – preventing health problems
- secondary – treating the health problems
- tertiary – maintenance or rehabilitation.

As a result, health services have been traditionally provided by primary care staff who provide the primary care (care delivered within a community setting, in the person's home or GP's surgery); this is often but not exclusively preventive care. Secondary care staff, who provide secondary and tertiary care (usually the treatment of individuals once they are suffering from a medically diagnosed condition or who are recovering from one). Secondary care has traditionally been delivered in hospital, care homes or similar settings; however, over the last 15 to 20 years, secondary care staff in the mental health field have also been working in community settings. In addition, services have traditionally been determined by professionals working within the health services. In more recent years, there has been a move to ensure that service users' needs are central to the process of determining mental health care. However, this is often hit and miss, with some good practices but many areas having limited service user involvement in this process.

DELIVERY TEAMS

In recent years, greater emphasis has been placed on knowledge, skills, experience and attitudes of health care providers rather than on traditional disciplines (Department of Health 2004a). However, most delivery teams are still mainly made up of a mixture of health and social care professions employed by the statutory services (National Health Service and Social Services), in other words 'professional groups'. Some of the most common delivery teams are briefly described below. The majority of them are usually made up of what are known as multidisciplinary teams (MDTs). The actual make-up of an MDT can vary due to the specific needs of the service users they serve (Wix & Humphreys 2005). Opie (1997) defines multidisciplinary working as something 'where members, operating out of their disciplinary bases, work parallel to each other, their primary objective being that of co-ordination'. In effect, this is the aim of MDTs.

PRIMARY HEALTH CARE

Primary health care can be defined as a community-based, point-of-contact health service comprising a range of services from health promotion and screening through to the diagnosis and treatment of medically diagnosed conditions provided by a range of community-based health services. This service is often the first point of contact for people with a mental illness.

MENTAL HEALTH IN-PATIENT UNITS/HOSPITALS

These are usually managed by a senior clinical nurse and staffed by mental health nurses, some of whom will have undertaken education and are registered nurses. Others have not taken professional education leading to registration but have had some training in the fundamentals of nursing care. Although not based on a ward, other professionals working in partnership with the nurses are medical staff, occupational therapists, psychologists and social workers (Ritter 1992). In recent years, acute in-patient care has been reformed (Department of Health 2002). There were several recommendations from the guidance, one being the way parts of mental health services interlock and communicate service users' needs. Specifically, the policy implementation guide recommends how in-patient care is to be organised and stresses the value of MDTs working together. These five professional groups mentioned above are considered by many to form the basis of an MDT and will be described in more detail later.

Within these are sub-areas specialising in the various defined areas that mental health problems are usually grouped under.

- Older adult (organic) – refers to people suffering mainly from reduced brain function and who in the later stages present with personality changes. People suffering from associated conditions are also prone to physical illness.
- Older adult (functional) – describes a group of people who are usually over 65 years of age and who suffer similar types of mental ill health as younger people, such as depression and psychosis.
- Day hospital – a service to help people of all ages, but more usually older adults, who need extra support from professionals through the day and have additional

support from carers or sometimes manage on their own (Muijen 1992). They offer a useful assessment and monitoring service as well as provision of treatment and can prevent relapse or arrange early in-patient care if needed.

- Rehabilitation – can be community- or institution-based. Community-based rehabilitation services often are a halfway house for people who are ready to leave 24-hour care but who still need some professional support. Institution-based care usually involves service users living with other service users, and yet they have their own personal space. Both approaches aim to achieve independent living by encouraging service users to manage their own day-to-day living, while still being supported by professionals.

- Acute mental health adult admission ward – this usually caters for people in their mid-teens to 65 years of age and deals with a wide range of mental health problems. Most acute wards are working towards single-sex provision. This is a result of female service users reporting actual or perceived sexual assaults, intimidation and feeling threatened by male service users, and the Government's policies concerning safety, privacy and dignity (Department of Health 2000a).

- Secure/forensic settings – the care setting will be medium- to high-security and will almost certainly be a locked environment. This setting is based in secondary mental health services and is responsible for service users whose offending behaviour has resulted from their being mentally ill or for those service users who are considered a severe danger to society.

- Psychiatric intensive care units (PICUs) – these were developed in Britain in the 1990s. Although there is no accepted, single definition, the various PICUs share common features. They have an intensive level of delivery of care by an MDT. Staffing levels are usually higher than general mental health in-patient facilities. They also tend to have more facilities such as garden areas, seclusion suites, activity and games room as well as quiet areas. Such units have a low level of security (Department of Health & Home Office 1992), which may be a locked area or lockable door of some form. Emphasis is placed on service users' mental health problems rather than on security.

COMMUNITY-BASED SERVICES

- Community mental health teams (CMHTs) – these can vary in the way they are set up but often have caseloads that specialise in certain age groups. Service users requiring this type of care will be receiving care from professionals working in secondary care but in a primary care setting, i.e. in the community.

- Assertive outreach (or community) teams – work with service users with severe mental health problems who have complex health and social care needs (Libberton 2000). Staff within the teams usually have smaller caseloads than those in CMHTs.

- Crisis-resolution (or home-support) teams – provide a 24-hour service to service users in their homes with the aim of avoiding hospital admission if at all possible and work towards the resolution of crises.

- Early-intervention teams – similar to crisis-resolution teams, these work specifically with service users who are showing the early symptoms of psychosis and try to reduce service users' longer-term dependency on services.
- Substance abuse/misuse services – although these have been placed under community-based services, in effect they can also be housed in in-patient units.
- Child and adolescent services – these services can also be in-patient based; however, many of these tend to work Monday to Friday with the service user returning to their home at weekends. The emphasis is on involving family members in the service users' care. There are also community-based services. Some are known as Child and Family Services as all tend to work with the family and not just the child or adolescent identified as having a mental health need.
- Prison in-reach – prisons in England and Wales are working with the NHS to introduce in-reach services, where NHS staff will work with prisoners to help treat their mental health problems.

OTHERS

Independent/private health providers

There are many large/small and national/local organisations that provide mental health care in the form of treatment centres and care homes. They range from secure environments to care homes.

Housing

Both local councils and private providers often have to work with people who have mental health problems. Mental health professionals frequently have to work with them to assist service users with their housing needs. Additionally, professionals have a role to educate housing personnel about mental health so they have a better understanding of service users' needs. The link between housing and mental health is clear; if it is not undertaken correctly, further problems can occur (Northmore 2001).

Education providers

Many people with mental health problems can benefit from learning new skills or knowledge. By working closely with health professionals, the learning can be undertaken without too much added stress. Health professionals can support the service users while undertaking the learning as well as educating the educators about mental illness and supporting them should any problems arise.

Leisure services

Exercise is known to help people to be not only physically healthier but also mentally healthier (Halliwell 2005). People who run or exercise often describe the 'high' achieved by the exercise. Not only will exercise help service users to enhance their self-esteem but may also help to reduce or maintain their weight. Some drugs used specifically for treating people with mental illness have been known to increase weight. Again, it is important for health professionals to work with staff in the leisure industry to educate and support them while they are working with service users.

Police

While the police do not provide health care, they do come into contact with people experiencing mental health problems. The police are often informed if an in-patient who is detained under the Mental Health Act 1983 leaves the in-patient unit without the knowledge or approval of health care professionals. The police will then attempt to find the missing person and return them to hospital. Additionally, the police can detain people they suspect of having a mental illness and who they believe are at risk to themselves or others.

Prison service

There are almost 80,000 people in prison in England and Wales (National Offender Management Service 2006). It has been suggested that 90% of prisoners have an identifiable mental illness; this figure rises to 95% in young offender prisons (Haines 2003). Sixty-six per cent of male prisoners and 55% of female prisoners have used illegal drugs in the previous year, compared to 13% males and 8% females in the general UK population (Wyatt 2004). Around 2% of remand prisoners attempt suicide each week (Haines 2003). The increase in prisoners with mental health problems over the last 10 to 15 years has had a major impact on English and Welsh prison life. Research of prison populations in England and Wales suggests that as much as one-third of prisoners had deliberately self-harmed at some point in their life (Maden 1994; Maden et al. 2000). Further, Shaw et al. (2003) clearly demonstrate that there has been a significant number of suicides in prisons. From April 2004, the NHS became responsible for the health of prisoners. All prison officers are given mental health awareness training and also receive training in self-harm and suicide prevention (Illingworth & Mabbett 2005).

Criminal justice workers (formerly probation officers)

With such a high proportion of prisoners suffering from mental illness, there is a need for mental health professionals to work in partnership with this agency. Criminal justice workers work to rehabilitate offenders by:

- enforcing the conditions of court orders and release licences
- conducting risk assessments of offenders to help minimise risk to the public
- ensuring offenders are aware of the impact of their crimes on their victims and the public.

Each year, criminal justice workers supervise over 200,000 offenders in Britain. They make assessments to advise courts, manage and enforce community orders and work with prisoners during and after sentencing. Criminal justice workers interact with offenders, victims, police and prison colleagues on a regular basis. They also work closely with:

- local authorities
- housing departments
- a range of statutory, independent and voluntary sector partners.

Youth offender teams (YOT)

Every local authority in England and Wales has a YOT. They are made up of representatives from the police, criminal justice services, and social, health, education, substance misuse and housing services. YOTs respond to the needs of young offenders in a far-reaching way as a result of multi-agency involvement. Each young offender is assessed with the use of a national assessment tool. (This is the Offender Assessment System, or OAS, a computerised tool internally developed by the Prison Service.) It identifies the specific problems that may make a young person offend and measures the risk they may cause to others.

ROLE(S) OF THE KEY PARTNERS

NON-PROFESSIONALS

Service users

The use of terminology is important as the term used may often affect how professionals and the general public view people with mental health problems. Although 'service user' is in vogue, there are negative connotations attached to it, for example when describing substance misusers. Additionally, it may imply a one-sided relationship and not a collaborative partnership between service users and service providers. The term 'patient' may also imply a passive role and is based on the recognition of pathology (Pilgrim & Rogers 1999). And many users do not view their problems in terms of illness (Barnham & Hayward 1991). The term 'consumer' has been used but has been rejected as a valid term because it implies that there is a choice in accepting services. However, Champ (2001) prefers the term because 'if he did not get the product offered he could complain, justifiably'; however, with some mental health service users this is not the case. The coercive nature of some people's compulsory detention in mental health services means that they are reluctant service users and are not exerting control over their service (Wilson 1995). Additionally, those entering hospital voluntarily often find there is little choice in the services offered (Pilgrim & Rogers 1999).

Since the late 1990s, Government guidelines have stated the need for service users to be central to health and social mental health care (Department of Health 1994, 1999b, 2001b). The Department of Health requires that NHS staff 'look at the provision of services from the patients' viewpoint and provide services that meet their reasonable expectations' (Department of Health 1999b) to make the service more responsive to service users' needs. One problem often stated as the reason why service users are not always included in service development is that traditional service delivery has been maintained by restrictive practice by professionals, to keep their own prestige and earnings. This is achieved by using professional jargon or shorthand – which, unless you are a professional you would not understand – and by long and costly training (Wilson 1995).

Many service users have reported on their experiences of mental health services, usually of in-patient care. Most, although not all, often recount negative experiences. However, not all service users hold this view. Maidment (2004) admits many have had bad experiences, and even admits to having had some herself. Nevertheless, she sees the care she received as, on the whole, good. It is worth noting that virtually all her positive examples are based on good communication and trusting relationships.

As service users are central to mental health care, it should go without saying that good communication between service users and mental health care staff is vital, and to achieve it there needs to be a level playing field between *all* parties. Yet Campbell (2000), when exploring his own mental illness and subsequent treatment, concludes that mental health care is based on inequality and that, instead of being central, service users are at the bottom of the pile.

Carers

It is important to remember that the needs of carers and the needs of service users are not always the same. Carers fulfil an important role for service users and the health service. Virtually every recent mental health policy acknowledges the important role of carers and asserts that they must be involved as full partners in the care package, (Department of Health 1998b, 1999a, 2000b, 2002; Sainsbury Centre for Mental Health 2001). However, that appears to not always be the case. 'What I notice the most about the care of people who are mentally ill is the fragmentation of it' (Chapman 2004). This statement was written by a carer and mother of a son in his 20s diagnosed as having severe and enduring paranoid schizophrenia. She adds that despite there being a value on 'joined-up multi-disciplinary care' each individual professional group either does not know what the other professionals are doing or disregards them. More worrying is her statement that some professionals find families (service users and carers) as nuisances. Yet there are many publications which clearly demonstrate that service users and carers are vital in the care process and that carers are often the 'glue that holds the system together' (Chapman 1997).

BENEFITS OF PARTNERSHIP WITH SERVICE USERS AND CARERS

It has been shown that involvement between service users, carers and professionals can lead to:

- mental health staff developing a better understanding of the effects of a severe mental illness on service users, their families and friends
- more effective partnerships and improved relationships between service users, carers and mental health professionals
- services being better targeted as they are based on service users' and carers' needs
- improved ways of meeting needs, e.g. enabling self-help and helping others in the community rather than being just receivers of care
- the views of service users and carers on the effectiveness of therapies being listened to (National Institute for Mental Health in England 2003b).

Charities, independent/voluntary and user groups

These groups play a very important role in the care of people with mental health problems. Although there are national voluntary and user groups, most people caring for those with mental health problems tend to use local groups as they are more responsive to their needs. These are very useful partners as they have often developed as a direct response to local need.

HEALTH AND SOCIAL CARE

PROFESSIONALS

From a professional viewpoint, key to delivering mental health care is the idea of multidisciplinary working, as discussed earlier. A mental health MDT is usually made up of a:

- nurse
- occupational therapist
- psychiatrist
- clinical psychologist
- approved social worker.

However, other disciplines (professional groups) or agencies can and do contribute on a regular basis, more often based on the individual service user's and/or carer's needs. To help in understanding this, what follows is a brief description of the roles of the main professional groups involved in providing mental health care.

Mental health nurses

Nurses are the largest single workforce in the NHS. There are 404,000 nurses qualified nurses, health visitors and midwives (Department of Health 2006). Registered mental health nurses have undertaken three years' education at a university from where they graduate and register as a nurse with the Nursing and Midwifery Council (NMC). They undertake continual professional development to help them meet the needs of service users (Nursing and Midwifery Council 2005). One key aspect of their role is to develop a trusting therapeutic relationship with service users. They use communication skills to help develop a rapport, which forms the basis of mental health nursing. Often further education is undertaken in specific therapies to enhance the therapeutic role. Nurses also administer medication and observe and report any improvements or side effects relating to the medication. Nurses undertake assessments of service users in order to identify their problems and needs; they then develop a plan of care in partnership with the service user. Following implementation of the interventions agreed in the plan of care, nurses evaluate the interventions and make adjustments to the plan or discontinue parts of it once they are no longer appropriate.

Occupational therapists (OTs)

OTs assess the physical, psychological and social functions of an individual, identify areas of dysfunction and involve the individual in a structured programme of activity to help overcome their dysfunction. The activities selected will relate to the service user's personal, social, cultural and economic needs and will reflect the environmental factors affecting their life (British Association/College of Occupational Therapists 2006). OTs can work in specialist areas and have distinct roles within that service, for example in forensic settings (Wix & Humphreys 2005).

Psychiatrists

Psychiatrists are doctors who have undertaken specialist training in mental health. As a result, they focus on diagnosing illnesses, prescribing treatments (often medication but could include other treatments such as electroconvulsive therapy), prognosis (predicting the outcome of an illness) and aetiology (trying to identify the cause of the illness). Historically, possibly owing to the medical education they receive, biological or physiological causations and their subsequent drug treatments have dominated psychiatrists' approach to treatment. In more recent years, psychiatrists have placed a greater emphasis on social and psychological factors, together with biological causes, and as a result they use psychological therapies as well as medication for their main treatment mode, although medication is still the primary mode of treatment.

General practitioners (GPs)

A GP is a doctor who provides primary care. A GP treats acute and chronic illnesses, provides preventive care and health education for all ages and both sexes. Some also care for hospitalised patients, do minor surgery and/or obstetrics. GPs can often be the first point of contact someone will have in the NHS when they need professional health care relating to a mental illness. One in four of GP consultations are with people who have mental health problems (Department of Health 2000b). For some, their GP will be the only person they come into contact with, but for others the GP may refer on to counsellors or nurses within the GP practice or for specialist mental health assessment and treatment from those members of the MDT working in secondary mental health care services. GPs can also refer to other agencies such as social services and clinical psychologists etc.

Approved social workers (ASW)

Under section 114 of the Mental Health Act 1983, a local social services authority must appoint a sufficient number of social workers who have 'appropriate competence in dealing with persons who are suffering from mental disorder'. Guidance is issued by the Central Council for Education and Training in Social Work as to the training which should be provided in order for social workers to fulfil this role. Most local authorities will ensure that an ASW is available 24 hours a day in order to make assessments in the community and thus to consider whether an application should be made for admission under the Act.

The Government was, until recently, planning major changes to the Mental Health Act – the law which enables people to be detained in hospital and be given treatment against their will (see Chapter Six of this book for a more detailed discussion). After a great deal of opposition to the proposed Bill from service users, carers and professionals, the Government has decided not to legislate the changes. However, elements of the changes that were to be included in the new Bill are still being proposed. The new amended Bill includes supervised treatment in the community to ensure that service users who have been discharged from compulsory treatment in hospital continue to comply with treatment. The proposals suggest that more groups of professionals than at present will have the ability to treat people without their consent.

Clinical psychologists

This is a relatively new professional group, which was first officially recognised with the foundation of the NHS in 1947 (Rogers and Pilgrim 2001). Clinical psychologists aim to reduce emotional suffering and to improve and promote mental health. They can treat a wide range of psychological problems, including anxiety, child and family problems, depression, relationship problems, as well as enduring mental illness. Clinical psychologists often carry out a clinical assessment using a range of methods, including psychometric tests, interviews and direct observation of behaviour. Following an assessment, a clinical psychologist will draw on psychological theory to put into words *why* a person is experiencing their specific symptoms and/or difficulties and, from this, identify a way to bring about improvement. The main therapies psychologists offer are:

- cognitive behavioural therapy (CBT) – looking at how thoughts, feelings and behaviours are all interconnected; this form of therapy is usually short term and problem-focused
- systemic therapy – how a 'problem' is created and maintained within a system (e.g. a family or couple); systemic therapists often see problems as being in a family rather than in a specific person
- psychodynamic therapy – focuses on early relationships in life (e.g. with parents/caregivers) and how these affect relationships in the present, leading to psychological distress (and therefore mental health problems); psychodynamic therapy examines repeated patterns of behaviour over a lifetime, and the psychodynamic therapist listens and tries to understand unconscious wishes, desires and conflicts
- behavioural therapy – based on the idea that all behaviour is learned through mechanisms of reinforcement; it therefore follows that behaviours can be unlearned (e.g. phobias, sexual problems).

Graduate mental health workers

These workers are a relatively new group of workers in the primary care team; officially they came into existence in 2004 and work closely with secondary care mental health staff (Department of Health/National Institute for Mental Health in England 2003). Their role has three main areas of focus:

1. face-to-face work with service users suffering from some of the common mental health problems, such as anxiety and depression
2. liaison with service users, carers and practice audit staff to establish and manage mental illness registers
3. liaison with the wider health and social care community, including police, criminal justice and non-government agencies who provide care and support to people experiencing mental health problems, to help ensure a seamless service.

Legal representative/advocate

Most legal representatives/advocates act on behalf of their client (service user) from the point of admission to discharge and afterwards. The whole process can be a major concern for some service users, especially if they have been detained under the Mental Health Act and are applying to a Mental Health Review Tribunal (Lee describes the role and function of the Mental Health Review Tribunal further in Chapter Six of this book). When service users have been detained, it is not uncommon for them to have concerns regarding specific aspects of their treatment and to sometimes wish to pursue complaints (formal or informal) about aspects of their care.

Owing to the nature of some service users' presenting symptoms, they are not always best able to speak up for themselves, in which case a legal representative or an advocate can represent them. Their role is often to act as a go-between to help enhance communication between the service user and the professionals. While most disputes are non-adversarial (in other words do not end up needing to go through the legal system), some do, in which case the legal representative or advocate may be required to act on the service user's behalf.

CONCLUSION

This chapter has introduced the idea of partnership working and its importance for effective partnership working in mental health care. Effective partnership work is necessary for the implementation of safe, sound and supportive mental health care (Department of Health 1998b). Partnership working depends on mutual respect and trust on the part of all partners. This may mean a change in some of the traditional power relationships between mental health professionals, service users and carers. In recent years, some of these traditional power relationships have been eroded. A greater emphasis on actively involving services users and carers in the development, delivery and evaluation of mental health care is possibly the best means of breaking down these power relationships and improving the effectiveness of mental health care provision.

REFERENCES

Audit Commission (1998) *A Fruitful Partnership: Effective Partnership Working.* London, Audit Commission.

Barnham P, Hayward R (1991) *From the Mental Patient to the Person.* London, Routledge.

Blane D (1991) Health professionals. In Scambler G (ed), *Sociology as Applied to Medicine* (3rd edn.). London, Bailliere Tindall, pp. 109–128.

British Association/College of Occupational Therapists (2006) Some key facts about occupational therapy, http://www.cot.org.uk/newpublic/otasacareer/what.php, accessed 11 July 2006.

Campbell P (2000) Challenging loss of power. In Read J, Reynolds J (eds), *Speaking Our Minds: An Anthology.* Basingstoke, Open University Press, pp. 56–62.

Campbell P (1997) Citizen Smith. *Nursing Times* **93**(41): 31–32.

Caplan G (1964) *Principles of Preventive Psychiatry.* New York, Basic Books.

Capon BJ (2005) *Panel Report from the Inquiry into the Care and Treatment of Richard King.* Norwich, Norfolk and Waveney Mental Health Partnership NHS Trust.

Champ S (2001) Keynote speech, 7th International Network for Psychiatric Nursing Research Conference (September, 2001). Royal College of Nursing, Oxford.

Chapman H (1997) Self-help groups, family carers and mental health. *Australian and New Zealand Journal of Mental Health Nursing* **6**(4): 148–155.

Chapman V (2004) Carer issues in mental health. In Kirby SD, Hart DA, Cross D, Mitchell G (eds), *Mental Health Nursing Competences For Practice*. Basingstoke, Palgrave Macmillan.

Coleman R, Harding E (2004) Can we really be partners? *Mental Health Nursing* **24**(5): 4–5.

Cook G, Gerrish K, Clarke C (2001) Decision-making in teams: issues arising from two UK evaluations. *Journal of Interprofessional Care* **15**(2): 141–151.

Department of Health (1990) HC90 23/LASL (90) *The Care Programme Approach for People with Mental Illness Referred to Specialist Psychiatric Services*. London, Her Majesty's Stationery Office.

Department of Health (1991) *Report on Confidential Enquiries in Maternal Death in the United Kingdom 1985–1987*. London, Her Majesty's Stationery Office.

Department of Health (1994) *Working in Partnership? A Collaborative Approach to Care: Report of the Mental Health Nursing Review Team*. London, Her Majesty's Stationery Office.

Department of Health (1998a) *Partnership in Action (New Opportunities for Joint Working between Health and Social Services): A Discussion Document*. London, Her Majesty's Stationery Office.

Department of Health (1998b) *Modernising Mental Health Services: Safe, Sound and Supportive*. London, Her Majesty's Stationery Office.

Department of Health (1999a) *National Service Framework for Mental Health: Modern Standards and Service Models*. London, Her Majesty's Stationery Office.

Department of Health (1999b) *Patient and Public Involvement in the New NHS*. London, Her Majesty's Stationery Office.

Department of Health (2000a) *Safer, Privacy and Dignity in Mental Health Units*. London, Her Majesty's Stationery Office.

Department of Health (2000b) *The NHS Plan*. London, Her Majesty's Stationery Office.

Department of Health (2001a) *Working Together – Learning Together: A Framework for Lifelong Learning for the NHS*. London, Her Majesty's Stationery Office.

Department of Health (2001b) *The Expert Patient*. London, Her Majesty's Stationery Office.

Department of Health (2002) *Mental Health Policy Implementation Guide: Adult Acute Inpatient Care Provision*. London, Her Majesty's Stationery Office.

Department of Health (2004a) *The NHS Knowledge and Skills Framework (NHSKSF) and the Development Review Process*. London, Her Majesty's Stationery Office.

Department of Health (2006) NHS staff 1995–2005, http://www.ic.nhs.uk/pubs/nhsstaff, accessed 18 July 2006.

Department of Health/Home Office (1992) *Review of Health and Social Services for Mentally Disordered Offenders and Others Requiring Similar Services* (Reed Report). London, Department of Health/Home Office.

Department of Health/National Institute for Mental Health in England (2003) *Fast Forwarding Primary Care Mental Health: Graduate Primary Care Mental Health Workers*. London, Department of Health.

Galvin SW, McCarthy S (1994) Multi-disciplinary community teams: clinging to the wreckage. *Journal of Mental Health* **3**: 167–174.

Goss S, Miller C (1995) *From Margin to Mainstream: Developing User- and Carer-centred Community Care*. York, Joseph Rowntree Foundation.

Haines G (2003) Developing the Health Care Workforce for London's Prisons. In *Workforce Matters*. London, Department of Health, p. 7.

Halliwell E (2005) *Up And Running? Exercise Therapy and the Treatment of Mild or Moderate Depression in Primary Care.* London, Mental Health Foundation.

Hudson B, Hardy B, Henwood M, Wistow G (1997) *Inter-Agency Collaboration: Final Report.* Leeds, Nuffield Institute for Health, Community Care Division.

Illingworth P, Mabbett A (2005) Prison officer entry level training (POELT): the new foundation course. *Prison Service Journal* January 2005 (157): 11–13.

Libberton P (2000) Getting your ACT together. *Mental Health Nursing* **20**(3): 14–17.

Lindow V (1991) Experts, lies and stereotypes. *The Health Service Journal.* **101**(5267): 18–19.

Lindow V (1996) Keynote address. Thriving, Not Surviving: Users' Needs in Mental Health Conference (29 March 1996) held at the Nuffield Institute for Health, University of Leeds.

Maden A (1994) A criminological and psychiatric survey of women serving a prison sentence. *British Journal of Criminology* **34**(2): 172–191.

Maden A, Chamberlain S, Gunn J (2000) Deliberate self-harm in sentenced male prisoners in England & Wales: some ethnic factors. *Criminal Behaviour & Mental Health* **10**(3): 199–204.

Maidment A (2004) User perspective – the good psychiatric nurse. In Kirby SD, Hart DA, Cross D, Mitchell G (eds), *Mental Health Nursing Competences For Practice.* Basingstoke, Palgrave Macmillan.

Mental Health Foundation (1994) *Creating Community Care.* London, Mental Health Foundation.

Millar B (2000) All in a day's work. *Therapy Weekly* **27**(10): 48.

Muijen MF (1992) Day care. In Brooking JI, Ritter SAH, Thomas BL (eds), *A Textbook of Psychiatric and Mental Health Nursing.* Edinburgh. Churchill Livingstone, pp. 313–322.

National Institute for Mental Health in England (2003a) *Cases for Change: A Review of the Foundations of Mental Health Policy and Practice 1997–2002.* London, Department of Health.

National Institute for Mental Health in England (2003b) *Cases for Change: User Involvement.* London, Department of Health.

Nursing and Midwifery Council (2005) *Nursing and Midwifery Council: The PREP Handbook.* London, Nursing and Midwifery Council.

National Offender Management Service (2006) Prison population and accommodation briefing, http://www.hmprisonservice.gov.uk/assets/documents/10001AE1Population Bulletin-Weekly31March2006.doc, accessed 6 July 2006.

Northmore S (2001) Improving partnership working in housing and mental health. In Balloch S, Taylor M (eds), *Partnership Working: Policy and Practice.* Bristol, The Policy Press.

Onyett S (2003) *Teamworking in Mental Health.* Basingstoke, Palgrave Macmillan.

Opie A (1997) Thinking teams, thinking clients: issues of discourse and representation in the work of health care teams. *Sociology of Health and Illness* **19**(3): 259–280.

Payne M (2000) *Teamwork in Mulitprofessional Care.* Basingstoke, Palgrave Macmillan.

Pietroni PC (1992) Towards reflective practice – the languages of health and social care. *Journal of Interprofessional Care* **6**(1): 7–16.

Pilgrim D, Rogers A (1999) *A Sociology of Mental Health and Illness.* Buckingham, Open University Press.

Repper J, Perkins R (2003) *Social Inclusion and Recovery: A Model for Mental Health Practice.* Edinburgh, Bailliere Tindall.

Ritchie J, Dick D, Lingham R (1994) *The Report of the Inquiry into the Care and Treatment of Christopher Clunis.* London, Her Majesty's Stationery Office.

Ritter SAH (1992) Organising inpatient care. In Brooking JI, Ritter SAH, Thomas BL (eds), *A Textbook of Psychiatric and Mental Health Nursing.* Edinburgh. Churchill Livingstone, pp. 295–311.

Rogers A, Pilgrim D (2001) *Mental Health Policy in Britain* (2nd edn.). Basingstoke, Palgrave Macmillan.

Ross F, Campbell F (1992) Interprofessional collaboration in the provision of aids for daily living and nursing equipment in the community – a district nurse and consumer perspective. *Journal of Interprofessional Care* 6(2): 109–118.

Sainsbury Centre for Mental Health (2001) *The Capable Practitioner.* London, Sainsbury Centre for Mental Health.

Shaw J, Appleby L, Baker D (2003) *A National Study of Prison Suicides 1999–2000. National Confidential Inquiry into Suicides and Homicides by People with Mental Illness.* Manchester, Department of Health.

Spokes K, Bond K, Lowe T, Jones J, Illingworth P, Brimbelcombe N, Wellman N (2002) HOVIS: The Hertfordshire/Oxford Violent Incident Study. *Journal of Psychiatric/Mental Health Nursing* 9(2): 199–209.

Stevenson O (1985) The community care of frail old people: co-operation in health and social care. *British Journal of Occupational Therapy* 48(9): 332–334.

Strauss G (1962) Tactics of lateral relationships: the purchasing agent. *Administrative Science Quarterly* September(7): 161–186.

Wilson G (1995) *Community Care – Ask the Service Users.* London, Chapman & Hall.

Wix S, Humphreys M (eds) (2005) *Multidisciplinary Working in Forensic Mental Health Care.* Edinburgh, Elsevier.

Wyatt J (2004) Improving the health of a captive population. *Health Management* 8(2): 14–16.

5 Promoting Mental Health

A. BROWNBILL AND S. CHELVANAYAGAM

Treating a disease by the time it is manifest is like starting to dig a well when you're dying of thirst. (Chinese proverb)

INTRODUCTION

The aim of this chapter is to provide an insight and understanding of mental health promotion. The role of mental health promotion is the prevention of mental health problems, the promotion of overall health and recovery and the reduction of discrimination and stigmatisation that people with mental health problems experience (Department of Health 1999a).

Often, health care practitioners appear to focus on illness and may see their role as one of removing illness or helping to control symptoms of illness. Health promotion can be more concerned with 'wellness'. Rather than asking the question about what diseases need to be eliminated or what symptoms need to be reduced, the question of what is required to stay well would be more pertinent. Instead of waiting for an illness to happen and then trying to fix it, health promotion is more about preventing that illness from happening in the first place or preventing a reoccurrence. These two branches of medicine, curative and preventive, have been related to the ancient Greek myths and in particular the two daughters of Asklepios – Panacea and Hygeia. Panacea relates to drugs and cures whereas Hygeia is more concerned with the environmental and preventive aspects of medicine (Waldron 1978, cited in Macdonald 1998). This approach prompts the question: 'What is wellness?' The World Health Organization's (WHO) definition of health as formulated in 1948 is:

Health is a state of complete physical, mental and social well-being and not merely the absence of disease or infirmity. (WHO, 1948)

Although this definition is frequently used, it does not acknowledge the links between physical, mental and social well-being in that they all have an effect on each other (Department of Health 2001; Lee & Chelvanayagam 2004).

Caring for Adults with Mental Health Problems   Edited by I. Peate and S. Chelvanayagam
© 2006 John Wiley & Sons, Ltd

BACKGROUND TO MENTAL HEALTH PROMOTION STRATEGY

The Government set one of its health targets as mental health services. This was because two of the most significant causes of poor health were mental health problems and coronary heart disease (Department of Health 1999b). On deciding to modernise mental health services, the Government developed the National Service Framework (NSF) for Mental Health (Department of Health, 1999a). The NSF contains seven standards regarding all aspects of mental health care. However, the first standard is concerned with mental health promotion (Table 5.1).

Table 5.1 Mental health promotion – Standard One of the NSF (Adapted from Department of Health 1999a)

Standard One: Mental Health Promotion

Aim: To ensure health and social services promote mental health and reduce the discrimination and social exclusion associated with mental health problems

Health and social services should:

- promote mental health for all, working with individuals and communities
- combat discrimination against individuals and groups with mental health problems, and promote their social inclusion.

WHAT IS MENTAL HEALTH PROMOTION AND HOW DOES IT WORK?

The Sainsbury Centre for Mental Health stipulates that:

Mental health promotion is essentially concerned with:

- how individuals, families, organisations and communities think and feel;
- the factors which influence how we think and feel individually and collectively;
- the impact this has on overall health and well-being (Sainsbury Centre for Mental Health 2005).

Therefore, mental health promotion is not solely to prevent mental illness and promote recovery from illness (although that is part of its remit) but also to focus on improving physical health and emotional resilience, tackling stigma and promoting social inclusion. It should include interventions to reduce stress at work, tackle bullying in schools and provide better environments and appropriate housing.

Mental health promotion also works at three levels that are all relevant to the whole population, individuals at risk (such as children growing up in a violent family environment), vulnerable groups (prisoners, asylum seekers, homeless people) and people with mental illnesses (Department of Health 2001).

Mental health promotion attempts to achieve its aims by:

strengthening individuals or increasing resilience by interventions designed to improve self-esteem and coping skills, such as communication skills or parenting skills

strengthening communities, which involves reducing stigma of mental illness so that individuals feel included (social inclusion), developing services that support people with mental illness within their communities, improving neighbourhood environments and supporting self-help groups

reducing structural barriers to mental health, which entails reducing discrimination and ensuring people with mental health problems have access to education, employment, housing and services.

In order to explore mental health promotion concepts, the following scenario will be used:

Scenario

Amy is 13 years old. She lives with her three siblings and parents, Mary and Joe, in a tower block of flats in a deprived and built-up area of the city. Her parents' relationship is very unstable: Joe is frequently violent towards Mary; Mary has left on several occasions. Mary has a history of depression. This means that when Mary is unwell, Amy (as the eldest child) has to care for her mother and siblings making sure the house is clean and there is food on the table for when her father comes home from work. Therefore, she is frequently late for school and is teased and bullied as her clothes are often dirty and ill-fitting. She struggles to keep up with her schoolwork because she is tired. Amy also has dyslexia. After school, Amy has to rush home and prepare the dinner and so has no time to play with her friends.

From this scenario it could be assumed that Amy is at risk of developing mental health problems now or later in life, and her mother Mary is at risk of suffering from a reoccurrence of her depressive illness. According to the Department of Health (2001), the factors which influence the development of mental health problems are categorised into five domains:

- individual risk factors
- family/social factors
- school context
- life events and situations
- community and cultural factors.

INDIVIDUAL RISK FACTORS

In the above scenario, the individual risk factors for Amy are her difficulties with her schoolwork and the insecure attachment she may have with Mary, due to her illness and the fact that Mary has left Joe on a number of occasions. Her attachment with her father Joe may be weak due to her fear of his violence (Heijmens Visser *et al.* 2000).

FAMILY/SOCIAL FACTORS

With respect to family factors, there is family violence and marital discord. For Amy's mother Mary, this violence will not only affect her physical health in respect of injuries but also have a detrimental effect on her mental state. People diagnosed with depression usually have a low self-esteem. The anger and violence directed towards her by Joe, her husband, will exacerbate her feelings of inadequacy making it more likely for a relapse in her mental state to occur. Children such as Amy and her siblings are exposed to this violence, which can result in psychological and physical health problems (Ramsay *et al.* 2002). In addition, Amy is neglected due to her mother's depressive illness and is socially isolated from her peer group due to having to care for her family.

SCHOOL CONTEXT

At school, Amy is bullied and has difficulty with her schoolwork. Evidence shows that bullying at school can be an indicator for mental health problems either currently or later in life (Wolke *et al.* 2000). Also, her difficulties with her schoolwork and her dyslexia may make it harder for her to achieve satisfactory grades in school; so her future employment opportunities will be limited. This would probably have long-term consequences for her quality of life.

LIFE EVENTS AND SITUATIONS

Amy is involved in caring for Mary and her family, which will create both a physical and psychological burden as she is unsupported by other family members or public services (Falkov 1998).

COMMUNITY AND CULTURAL FACTORS

Amy lives in a socially deprived area; socially deprived areas, it has been demonstrated, can contribute to poor mental health (Dalgard & Tambs 1997). In addition, owing to her domestic environment, Amy does not have a competent role model to demonstrate the use of effective coping strategies. Her father uses violence to demonstrate his distress; her mother, owing to her illness, has difficulty articulating her feelings and emotions. Finally, owing to mental health problems and their socio-economic situation, Amy and her family may face discrimination and be stigmatised by the public and public services (Department of Health 2002; Crisp 1998).

NEEDS ASSESSMENT OF AMY AND HER FAMILY

Initially, mental health practitioners would be required to undertake a needs assessment in order to ascertain what could be done to prevent Amy and her siblings from developing mental illnesses and to help promote recovery from illness for Mary, Amy's mother. A thorough assessment of needs is often overlooked, and health practitioners will sometimes carry out health promotion activities without fully understanding what the needs are. Often, when assessing, health practitioners will tend to concentrate on needs, deficits or weaknesses. It has been found to be important not just to assess needs but also to assess the strengths, skills and resources available within individuals and communities. Red Cross Publications (2004) note that 'human capital' (knowledge, skills, health, education, physical ability) determine an individual's resilience more than any other asset.

The term 'health needs' can be considered from a variety of viewpoints. Bradshaw (1972) notes that there are four types of need:

- normative
- felt
- expressed
- comparative.

Naidoo and Wills (2000) explain these needs further. A *normative* need would be a need that had been decided by health care practitioners. Normative needs are not always the same as the needs that service users might say they have. For practitioners to decide that there is a normative need could be considered to be a paternalistic approach to needs assessment as it is their own subjective belief and is not necessarily the client's need.

An example of a normative need is if a health care practitioner saw that Mary was having difficulty coping with Joe and caring for her family and was becoming increasingly more depressed the health care practitioner may decide that Mary had a *need* for greater resilience.

If Mary herself felt or believed that she had difficulties in coping, this would be considered a *felt* need.

Once Mary had expressed her difficulties with coping to the health care practitioner, it would become an *expressed* need. It can be useful to think of this in more detail. Felt needs are not always expressed. A person who feels that they are not coping well with life may be reluctant to express this for fear of being considered weak and needy, or in Mary's case she may fear further abuse from Joe should he discover her disclosure. Mary may become concerned at needing to involve health care practitioners and worried about the consequences of being labelled as having a mental illness. There is much stigma associated with being thought of as dependent, and so people may try to hide the fact that they are not coping. Language difficulties and cultural factors may also prevent disclosure of a perceived need.

Comparative needs may be thought to be about equity. If two people or two groups of people with the same need are treated differently, that is inequitable. According to the *Independent Inquiry into Inequalities in Health* report (Acheson 1998), equity is a founding principle of the NHS and is central to Government policy.

Health promotion needs can be assessed in a variety of ways including:

- individual interviews
- questionnaires
- comparison with other similar groups in society
- health care practitioner observations.

The health care practitioner's own observations of the service user's demeanour and behaviour can give much information about how the service user feels about themselves but this can also be compromised by the health care practitioner's subjectivity. With Amy and her family, the health care practitioner would need to consider which assessment tools would be most appropriate in the circumstances. For example, is it appropriate to interview Amy or Mary together or separately? How ethical would it be to consult Amy's teachers at school? Should Joe be interviewed or will that put Mary at greater risk of further abuse?

From a needs assessment, it could be ascertained that Amy and her family may require mental health promotion interventions in the following areas:

- improving emotional resilience
- promoting recovery
- tackling stigma
- promoting social inclusion and challenging inequality.

IMPROVING EMOTIONAL RESILIENCE

'Resilience' is defined as 'the ability of an ecosystem to return to its original state after being disturbed' (Makins 1991). It may be thought of as the ability to recover easily and quickly from shock, illness or hardship, for example. It derives from the Latin *resilire* – to jump back. It could be considered to be the psychosocial equivalent of the immune system. Being inoculated against diseases increases our own natural resistance and thereby reduces the chances of our developing that particular illness. There are no vaccinations against any of the mental illnesses; however, there is an appropriate analogy in that, as in physical illnesses where exposure to disease can make people more resistant, in mental health it is noted that resilience can be increased by being exposed to difficult situations so that coping strategies can be developed. People can develop their own resilience to life's complex situations by giving themselves the opportunities to face new challenges. Hechtman's (1991) research on resilience in children diagnosed with attention deficit disorder demonstrates that the following factors seem to be important in developing resilience:

- absence of health problems
- positive temperament factors and activity
- social responsiveness
- higher-than-average intelligence
- positive self-esteem
- autonomy
- good peer relationships.

Factors that help to make children more resilient, according to Jacelon (1997), include:

- secure attachments and affection from others
- positive attitude
- good communication skills
- at least one good parent–child relationship
- supervision and discipline from carers and teachers
- wider supportive network, e.g. caring grandparents
- school with positive policies on key issues, such as bullying
- good standard of living.

With regard to some of the qualities that seem to promote resilience, Maslow's 'hierarchy of needs' addresses some of these in his sections on the need to belong, to have relationships and the need for self-esteem, which includes confidence, competence, mastery and independence (Townsend 2000; Boeree 1998).

PROMOTING RECOVERY

The concept of 'recovery' was introduced by those who had experienced mental health problems rather than by mental health practitioners (Allott *et al.* 2002). There has been much expressed concern by people who experience mental illness that the term 'recovery' implies 'cure'. Therefore, once the person with mental illness is seen as 'recovered' the services and help they depend on to maintain their health will be removed because they are 'cured' (Beresford & Hopton 2003). Essentially, recovery is seen as part of a process that includes the person with mental illness being empowered to take an active role in managing their mental health while also managing day-to-day life, living independently and contributing to society (Allott *et al.* 2002). To achieve this process, a health care practitioner needs to work with the person with a mental illness by helping them to make decisions about their illness and their everyday needs by empowering them with relevant information and emotional support. In addition, the focus should be on wellness and positive mental health.

In relation to the earlier scenario, to promote Mary's recovery the health care practitioner would initially need to elicit from Mary her understanding of her illness and treatment. For example, Mary may need information about depression and accessing help and treatment. She may have never disclosed to her general practitioner that she suffers from low mood and therefore may never have received treatment. Alternatively, Mary may be receiving appropriate medical treatment, such as antidepressant therapy, but may also require psychological interventions, such as counselling, to help her develop coping strategies to manage her illness and her lifestyle. (see Chapter 14 of this book). Mary may also accept some assistance with cooking, cleaning and shopping when she is unwell, which will mean that Amy will no longer have to fulfil these duties. Mary may also need information and advice regarding domestic violence in order for her to make a decision about her relationship with Joe. She may decide that she will discuss her concerns with Joe and request that they consider relationship counselling. In addition, people who experience mental illness report that peer support or self-help organisations are key components to the recovery process (Mead & Copeland 2000). This would entail the health care practitioner providing Mary with details of self-help organisations or groups, such as support groups for women who experience depression or domestic violence. It may mean that initially Mary may benefit from her health care practitioner accompanying her to such meetings. It is anticipated that increased education and awareness with appropriate treatment and support would promote Mary's recovery. In addition, Mary's recovery would relieve Amy of the household chores, which have had a deleterious effect on her psychological, physical and social functioning.

TACKLING STIGMA

'Stigma' is defined as 'a mark of disgrace or discredit that sets a person side from others' (Byrne 2001). Mental illness is widely reported as a stigmatising condition (Byrne 2001). Although mental illness can affect one in six people during their lifetime, people still view mental illness with fear, hostility and disapproval (Changing Minds 2006). Changing Minds was a campaign developed by the Royal College of Psychiatrists that aimed to reduce the stigma of mental illness. As well as completing a national survey to ascertain people's perceptions of different types of mental illness, it provides a range of easily accessible information about mental illness (Crisp et al. 2000). The survey discovered that the general population has negative opinions about people with mental illnesses. In particular, it was reported that people with schizophrenia were perceived as dangerous and people with eating disorders were felt to have self-inflicted illnesses. In addition, the general opinion was that people with any form of mental illness were difficult to talk to, were perceived as different and were believed to be unpredictable (Crisp et al. 2000).

Therefore, owing to the stigma surrounding mental illness and the belief that people with depression should 'pull themselves together' (Semple et al. 2005), Mary may be reluctant to seek help for fear of humiliation and may be reluctant for health care practitioners to visit her at home. If Mary does not seek help for her depressive illness, her condition may deteriorate and she may attempt self-harm (see Chapter 8 in this book). Amy will continue with shopping, cleaning, cooking and looking after her siblings to the extent that she may become physically and psychologically unwell. Amy may be reluctant to inform teachers at her school of her mother's health as she may be frightened that her mother will be taken into hospital. Therefore, it is important to discuss with Mary the importance of accessing help and treatment, not purely to treat her depressive illness but also to prevent further deterioration of her condition to the extent that admission to a mental health unit is required, which may exacerbate Mary's concerns regarding stigmatisation.

The media, specifically the tabloid press, has been blamed for its negative portrayal of mental illness, in particular its initial coverage of a famous boxer's detention in a mental health unit (Clarke 2004). The headline ran was 'BONKERS BRUNO LOCKED UP' (The Sun 23 September 2003), which was quickly retracted following a public outcry. However, organisations such as MIND and SANE, who provide information and advice on mental illness, have helped to counteract some of this negative media coverage by directly responding to inappropriate messages and challenging many beliefs based on ignorance or prejudice rather than fact.

Education concerning mental illness is now being incorporated into the school curriculum in the hope that the next generation will gain knowledge and an understanding about mental health issues and also that children in Amy's situation are aware that there is help, treatment and support.

PROMOTING SOCIAL INCLUSION AND TACKLING INEQUALITY

Only 15% of people with serious mental health problems are employed; those experiencing mental health problems are one of the most excluded groups in society (Evans & Repper, 2000). People who use mental health services are likely to be poor, unemployed, living in poor accommodation and isolated (Sainsbury Centre for Mental Health 2002).

As described above, people with mental health problems frequently endure stigma and discrimination. Employers are reluctant to employ people with mental health problems despite the Disability Discrimination Act 1995, which stipulates that it is unlawful to discriminate against disabled people in employment, provision of goods, services, transport and education (Community Legal Services Direct 2006).

People with mental health problems have difficulty accessing the services they require, such as housing and transport. Educational and leisure facilities are only now beginning to offer benefits, such as reducing the cost of gym membership, to people with mental health problems. Helliwell (2005) shows that physical exercise is an effective treatment for depression.

Social exclusion is defined as:

> Social exclusion happens when people or places suffer from a series of problems such as unemployment, discrimination, poor skills, low incomes, poor housing, high crime, ill health and family breakdown. When such problems combine they can create a vicious cycle (Social Exclusion Unit 2006)

The Social Exclusion Unit was established to tackle issues of stigmatisation, discrimination and social inequality. The aim of programmes devised by the Social Exclusion Unit are to develop policy, strategy and practice so that users have equal opportunities to engage in everyday life (Sainsbury Centre for Mental Health 2002). The Social Exclusion Unit's action plan includes:

- tackling discrimination and stigma
- employment opportunities that reflect people's expertise
- supporting families
- access to appropriate housing, financial advice and transport.

Returning to the scenario, the definition of 'social exclusion' reflects Amy and her family's situation: they live in a socially deprived area, and this can have detrimental effects on their mental health. Mary is suffering from depression and marital disharmony, which in itself may lead to isolation. Social isolation can detrimentally affect Mary's mental state, and this may lead to self-harm or even suicide. Amy, as her mother's carer, needs support, not only help with household chores but also the opportunity to discuss her concerns about her family with health care practitioners and other teenagers in a similar situation. Amy is isolated as she does not have time to meet her friends due to her carer role. Amy may also feel disadvantaged due to her dyslexia and tiredness making it difficult for her to keep up with her schoolwork.

Access to educational, leisure and employment opportunities with support from a health care practitioner may help to improve Mary's mental state, provide her with a range of skills and help her achieve paid employment.

METHODS AND APPROACHES

As with the assessment of health promotion needs and strengths, there are a few different ways of thinking about methods, approaches or strategies to achieving mental well-being. Naidoo and Wills (2000) consider five different approaches:

1. medical or preventive
2. behavioural change
3. educational
4. empowerment
5. social change.

The Ottawa Charter for Health Promotion (WHO 1986) suggests five strategies:

- building healthy public policy
- creating supportive environments

- strengthening community actions
- developing personal skills
- reorienting health services.

The *Circle of Health* (Prince Edward Island Health and Community Services Agency 1996) uses these five strategies within an overall framework that can be of help in thinking about how to go about planning health promotion interventions. Many practitioners in mental health settings will probably not become too involved in reorganising health services, building healthy public policy or bringing about changes at a societal level. There may be occasions where practitioners are involved in community actions as part of initiatives such as World Mental Health Day. This work can often have a good effect in enabling current users of mental health services to educate the general public about mental illness, thereby promoting access to services, creating opportunities for more discussion and reducing stigma. There may also be times when mental health workers feel sufficiently motivated to try to bring about policy changes by lobbying their representatives on committees and making representations to Members of Parliament. However, their key focus would consist of working with individuals and small groups of users of mental health services in order to provide education and to support them in developing personal skills so as to promote their health.

The behavioural change approach is concerned with helping people to make the changes that would lead to a healthier lifestyle. Recent emphasis on reducing smoking and changing diets are good examples of this in relation to physical health primarily; however, the links between physical health and mental health are so clear that interventions to improve one area of our lives will have a direct effect on other areas. The educational approach is often the most popular method used in health promotion even though it is questionable to what extent knowledge has an impact on behaviour: for example, although all packets of cigarettes and tobacco draw attention to health risks, some people still choose to continue to smoke. However, education is important, as people are enabled to make informed choices about their lifestyle. It is important to note that education is part of empowerment. If Amy were to be educated about some of the support systems available with regard to being bullied, she may then be empowered to take advantage of services available.

EVALUATION OF MENTAL HEALTH PROMOTION INTERVENTIONS

'Health promotion is as much about processes and ways of working as the content and outcome of programmes' (Naidoo & Wills 1998). Evaluation is attributing value to an intervention by gathering reliable and valid information about it in a systematic way, and by making comparisons (Øvretveit 1998). It consists of establishing the outcome of a treatment or health promotion strategy. Although it is the last step in the process, it needs to be considered when planning a project as it has to determine whether a programme is effective. To do this, a measurement needs to be taken before a strategy is implemented that can be repeated on completion of the health promotion activity and compared with the initial measurement to see if any learning or improvements had occurred.

Health practitioners need to know whether interventions work in order to improve their knowledge. This knowledge helps to provide information to service users about different options. Evaluation can also help health practitioners understand how initiatives have worked and how any knowledge gained can be transferred to other situations or service users groups, and it helps to ensure that resources are used efficiently (Naidoo & Wills 2000). In considering different types of evaluation, it is valuable to address the following points as described by Nagy and Fawcett (2006):

- Efficacy: Does it work?
- Explanation: Why and how does it work?
- Outcomes: What are all the effects?
- Outcomes sustained: How long do the effects last?
- Resources used: What does it cost?
- Acceptability, satisfaction: What do clients think about it?
- Equity: Can everybody benefit from it?
- Development: Can we improve it?

According to Naidoo and Wills (2000), evaluation can also be divided into three areas:

1. process evaluation
2. impact evaluation
3. outcome evaluation.

Process evaluation is concerned with looking at the health promotion methods used and how the participants responded to the methods. Impact evaluation is concerned with the immediate effects of the activity, whereas outcome evaluation is focused on the longer-term results (outcome) of the strategy and therefore on how successful the strategy was in making an effective change occur. For example, if a programme designed to promote social inclusion was implemented with Amy, the process evaluation would ask Amy questions about how much she enjoyed the activity. Which parts were most useful? What was the most difficult aspect? Should anything be omitted or should anything else be introduced? The impact evaluation would ask the question 'To what extent has social inclusion been increased soon after the activity?' The outcome evaluation would ask for how long the changes had been sustained.

CONCLUSION

In conclusion, the Department of Health (2001) has stated that mental health promotion can:

- improve physical health and well-being
- prevent or reduce the risk of some mental health problems
- assist recovery from mental health problems
- improve mental health services and the quality of life for people experiencing mental health problems
- strengthen the capacity of communities to support social inclusion, tolerance and participation, and reduce vulnerability to socio-economic stresses
- improve the mental health literacy of individuals, organisations and communities
- improve health at work, increasing productivity and reducing sickness and absence.

This chapter has aimed to provide an insight into the complex area of mental health promotion. It is important to realise that the cost of illness is immeasurable both in monetary terms and human cost; however, prevention of illness saves costs to Government spending but most importantly to a person's quality of life, which is priceless.

REFERENCES

Acheson D (1998) *Independent Inquiry into Inequalities in Health.* London, The Stationery Office.

Allott P, Loganathan L, Fulford KWM (2002) Discovering hope for recovery from a British perspective: a review of a selection of recovery literature, implications for practice and systems change. *Canadian Journal of Community Mental Health* **21**(2): 13–34.

Beresford P, Hopton J (2003) Recovery or independent living? *Openmind* **124**: 16–17.

Boeree CG (1998) *Abraham Maslow 1908–1970,* http://www.ship.edu/~cgboeree/maslow. html, accessed 6 July 2006.

Bradshaw J (1972) *The Concept of Social Need.* London, New Society.

Byrne P (2001) Psychiatric stigma. *British Journal of Psychiatry* **178**: 281–284.

Changing Minds (2006) Mental Disorders: challenging prejudices, http://www.rcpsych. ac.uk/campaigns/changingminds/whatisstigma/mentaldisorderschallenging.aspx, accessed 12 July 2006.

Clarke J (2004) Mad, bad and dangerous: the media and mental illness *Mental Health Practice* **7**(10): 16–19.

Community Legal Services Direct (2006) Rights for disabled people, http://www.clsdirect. org.uk/documents/18-Disabilities(FILECOPY).pdf, accessed 13 July 2006.

Crisp A (1998) Changing minds: every family in the land: the coming college campaign to reduce the stigmatisation of those with mental health problems. *Bulletin of the Royal College of Psychiatrists* **22**: 328–329.

Crisp AH, Gelder MG, Rix S, Meltzer HI, Rowlands GJ (2000) Stigmatisation of people with mental illness. *British Journal of Psychiatry* **177**: 4–7.

Dalgard OS, Tambs K (1997) Urban environment and mental health: a longitudinal study *British Journal of Psychiatry* **171**(July): 530–536.

Department of Health (2002) *Developing services for carers and families of people with mental illness*. London, Department of Health.

Department of Health (2001) *Making it Happen: A guide to delivering mental health promotion*. London, Department of Health.

Department of Health (1999a) *Modern Standards and Service Models: Mental Health, National Service Framework*. London, Department of Health.

Department of Health (1999b) *Saving Lives: Our Healthier Nation*. London, Department of Health.

Evans J, Repper J (2000) Employment, social inclusion and mental health. *Journal of Psychiatric and Mental Health Nursing* **7**(1): 15–24.

Falkov A (1998) *Crossing Bridges*. London, Department of Health.

Hechtman L (1991) Resilience and vulnerability in long-term outcome of ADHD. *Canadian Journal of Psychiatry* **36**(6): 415–421.

Heijmens Visser J, van der Ende J, Koot HM, Verhulst FC (2000) Predictors of psychopathology in young adults referred to mental health services in childhood or adolescence. *British Journal of Psychiatry* **177**(July): 59–65.

Helliwell E (2005) *Up And Running? Exercise therapy and the treatment of mild or moderate depression in primary care*. London, Mental Health Foundation.

Jacelon CS (1997) The trait and process of resilience. *Journal of Advanced Nursing* **25**(1): 123–129.

Lee S, Chelvanayagam S (2004) *Mental Health Promotion Needs Analysis: A Report for St Albans and Harpenden Primary Care Trust Part II*. Hatfield, University of Hertfordshire.

Macdonald TH (1998) *Rethinking Health Promotion: A Global Approach*. London, Routledge.

Makins M (ed) (1991) *Collins English Dictionary* (3rd edn.). Glasgow, HarperCollins.

Mead S, Copeland ME (2000) What recovery means to us. *Community Mental Health Journal* **36**(3): 325–328.

Naidoo J, Wills J (1998) *Practising Health Promotion. Dilemmas and Challenges*. London, Bailliere Tindall.

Naidoo J, Wills J (2000) *Health Promotion: Foundations for Practice* (2nd edn.). London, Harcourt.

Nagy J, Fawcett SB (2006) *Community Toolbox: Our Evaluation Model: Evaluating Comprehensive Community Initiatives*. Lawrence, KS, University of Kansas.

Øvretveit J (1998) *Evaluating Health Interventions*. Buckingham, Open University Press.

Prince Edward Island Health and Community Services Agency (1996) *Circle of Health*. Charlottetown, Canada, The Quaich, Inc.

Ramsay J, Richardson J, Carter YH, Davidson LL, Feder G (2002) Should health professionals screen women for domestic violence? Systematic review. *British Medical Journal* **325**(7359): 314–318.

Red Cross Publications (2004) From risk to resilience: helping communities cope with crisis. World Disasters Report 2004, http://www.ifrc.org/publicat/wdr2004/chapter1.asp, accessed 6 July 2006.

Sainsbury Centre for Mental Health (2002) *An Executive Briefing on 'Working for Inclusion'*. London, Sainsbury Centre for Mental Health.

Sainsbury Centre for Mental Health (2005) *Mental Health Promotion – Implementing Standard One of the National Service Framework for Mental Health.* London, Sainsbury Centre for Mental Health.

Semple D, Smyth R, Burns J, Darjee R, McIntosh A (2005) *Oxford Textbook of Psychiatry.* Oxford, Oxford University Press.

Social Exclusion Unit (2006) What is social exclusion? http://www.socialexclusionunit. gov.uk/page.asp?id=213, accessed 13 July 2006.

Townsend MC (2000) *Psychiatric Mental Health Nursing; Concepts of Care* (3rd edn.). Philadelphia, FA Davis.

Wolke D, Woods S, Bloomfield L, Karstadt L (2000) The association between direct and relational bullying and behaviour problems among primary school children. *Journal Child Psychology and Psychiatry, and Allied Disciplines* **41**(8): 989–1002.

World Health Organization (1986) *Ottawa Charter: First International Conference on Health Promotion.* Geneva, World Health Organization.

World Health Organization (1948) Preamble to the Constitution of the World Health Organization as adopted by the International Health Conference, New York, 19–22 June, 1946, http://www.who.int/about/definition/en/, accessed 6 July 2006.

6 Legal Matters

S. LEE

INTRODUCTION

This chapter intends to provide a brief overview of some of the legislation that affects mental health practice and the lives of the users of mental health services. Readers should note that the author's background is in mental health practice and the content of this chapter does not intend to provide legal interpretations of the legislation under discussion. It is not possible to detail all aspects of every piece of legislation; the aim is to raise awareness of the key issues that may impact on mental health care.

Those who are involved in the care of people with mental health problems should not only practise within the legal framework but also aim to provide good care at all times. In many ways, legislation – Acts of Parliament – affects all our lives. For example, right of access to one's own physical and mental health records is subject to the Access to Health Record Act 1990; entitlement to welfare benefits is governed by social security laws and the detention of mentally ill people in hospital is regulated by the current Mental Health Act 1983 (MHA 1983).

Readers should note that there is separate mental health legislation for Scotland and Northern Ireland. For the purpose of this chapter, the MHA 1983 for England and Wales will be addressed; this Act exerts great influence on mental health practice. Other key pieces of legislation that may impact on mental health care are:

- The Disability Discrimination Act (DDA)1995
- The Human Rights Act (HRA) 1998
- The Mental Incapacity Act (MIA) 2005.

The impact of some of the legislation on mental health service users can be profound for a variety of reasons. Service users may find themselves in a perpetual cycle of poverty as the welfare benefit system limits the amount of income that can be earned while claiming state benefits. The system appears to fail to provide the flexibility of facilitating a back-to-work initiative in a sufficient manner. Stopping and reclaiming benefits can be a daunting task, and the time it takes for benefits to be reinstated might render the user without money for a short time. Hence, while

Caring for Adults with Mental Health Problems   Edited by I. Peate and S. Chelvanayagam
© 2006 John Wiley & Sons, Ltd

some legislation may have a protective or therapeutic element, other legislation could also have a perverse effect.

The Government announced in March 2006 its decision not to proceed with the proposed Mental Health Bill; however, an amendment to the 1983 Act will be made instead. Some aspects of the proposal had been subject to intense debate and lobbying as it was felt that this may not have been in the best interest of mentally ill people. The tension between civil liberty and the rights of mentally ill people and public safety as a result of risk behaviour continues to be a highly charged debate by society as a whole.

For those admitted to hospital with a mental health problem, it is important that carers are fully aware of the two categories of mental health service users: those generally known as informal or voluntary admission patients and those who are admitted under a compulsory detention order of the MHA 1983. Those admitted informally or voluntarily are those who have agreed or consented to the admission taking place and accept treatment. However, individuals have the right to withdraw consent or refuse treatment after admission at any time. They are not subject to the provisions of the MHA 1983. Reflecting their informal status, the service user may decide to leave hospital at their own will and at any time. Good practice suggests that informal admission which represents the least restrictive option should always be considered before compulsory detention is contemplated. Staff should be aware of the distinction between discharge from hospital and discharge from detention. Individuals may agree to remaining in hospital and accepting treatment while being an informal patient. Hence, discharging from detention does not necessarily mean leaving hospital.

IMPLEMENTING THE MHA 1983

When service users are admitted under a compulsory detention order of the MHA 1983, this implies that admission has taken place without the expressed agreement or consent of the individual concerned. There is an obligation for practitioners to observe the requirements of the MHA 1983. In addition, there is also an obligation to follow the guidance set out in the *Code of Practice* (Department of Health 1999a). Although the MHA 1983 'does not impose a legal duty to comply with the Code . . . failure to follow it could be referred to in evidence in legal proceedings' (Department of Health 1999a). The *Code of Practice* has been prepared in accordance with section 118 of the MHA 1983; hence, it has the status of 'a statutory document' (Department of Health 1999a).

It is recommended that carers familiarise themselves with the associated sections of the Act as well as the *Code of Practice* prior to and on each occasion when dealing with a compulsory detention order. In this way, the practitioner is able to apply the detail in the Act in an appropriate and legal way as well as implementing good practice in an informed manner, in response to specific needs. Learning is more meaningful when the knowledge gained is related to the specific circumstance.

The Act is written in legal language and implementing it can be complex. A great deal of interpretation of the Act has been made by the courts leading to a substantive body of case law (Lee & Warrener 2005). Readers should refer to the *Mental Health Act Manual* (Jones 2004) for specific details of the sections associated with a detention order. There are occasions when aspects of the service user's circumstances are such that other legislation applies while detained under a result of the MHA 1983. For example, staff must comply with the relevant Articles of the Human Rights Act 1998 (Her Majesty's Stationery Office, 1998) when caring for those in their care.

Applying the MHA 1983 in practice requires multi-professional and multi-agency cooperation. Most mental health service providers have set up specific multi-agency fora for the purpose of the MHA 1983. These fora concern general practitioners (GPs), approved social workers (ASWs), police, the service user's family and hospital staff. It is important to have in place clear local policies and procedures for each of the staff groups to follow, as well as a joint training approach in order that each group understands each other's role. Regular meetings and reviews by the multi-agency fora foster good working relationships, which works towards the MHA 1983 being implemented smoothly and legally at an operational level.

For example, section 136 empowers police officers to remove a person who appears to be mentally disordered to a place of safety for the purpose of a mental health assessment. There needs to have been agreed a designated place of safety to where the police can bring the person. The procedure for securing attendance by appropriate personnel (psychiatric medical practitioner and ASWs) to carry out the assessment should have been in place for the police officers to act upon. Joint training for all the parties concerned would enable an understanding and discussion of each other's role.

MHA 1983 FOR ENGLAND AND WALES

For all admissions to hospital under the MHA 1983, there are specific procedures that must be adhered to in order that the admission becomes legal; these include having the correct official paperwork completed as dictated in the Act. There are also duties that must be carried out by practitioners and the hospital concerned in order that the various requirements of the Act are fulfilled. For example, the service user must be informed of their rights while under detention, and the hospital has a duty to inform the nearest relative of the admission.

The MHA 1983 is primarily concerned with people who are deemed mentally disordered and who require admission to hospital under a compulsory detention order. The MHA 1983 is divided into various parts; there are four main regulatory functions associated with the Act:

- admission procedure to hospital
- treatment and the lives of service users while under detention in hospital

- rights and protection of service users while detained in hospital
- provision of after-care when discharged from detention.

Part I of the MHA deals with the definitions of mental disorder and the categories of mental disorder. The categories are:

- mental illness
- mental impairment
- severe mental impairment
- psychopathic disorder.

One or more of the above categories must be met when admission to hospital under compulsory detention is necessary. The Act specifically excludes admission to hospital solely on the grounds that the individual is promiscuous or involved in other immoral conduct, considered as sexually deviant or dependent on alcohol or drugs. It cannot be applied to people suffering from a physical illness. In general, the grounds for detention are in the interest of the person's health or safety or with a view to the protection of others.

Part II of the Act sets out the admissions for civil detention. The responsible medical officer (RMO) who is the nominated consultant psychiatrist in charge of the service user's treatment may discharge the detained person at any time from detention. When working in a hospital setting, mental health staff are most likely to come across are sections 2, 3, 4 and 5. Service users may be admitted for assessment or assessment followed by treatment (section 2), this section cannot be renewed; or treatment (section 3) when individuals are subject to provisions of Part IV of the Act, which regulates aspects of the treatment. Section 3 may last up to six months and can be renewed. The RMO may grant leave of absence to a detained patient under section 17; staff must be fully aware of the conditions attached to the leave granted.

The provisions in section 4 facilitate emergency admissions. Section 5 deals with service users already in hospital informally when they present a particular risk and satisfy the definition of mental disorder; it empowers a medical practitioner or a nurse of a certain qualification to hold the individual for a specific length of time. Occasionally, staff may come across section 7 (guardianship order), which enables individuals to receive community care under an authoritative framework. A guardian who may be the local authority or a named individual is appointed; the powers of the guardian are set out in the *Code of Practice* (Department of Health 1999a). In general, guardianship is used when dealing with people who have a mental disorder and lack the capacity (usually learning disability or dementia) to consent to care but do not require hospital treatment. Guardianship represents the least restrictive alternative for this group of service users.

Part III of the Act refers to people admitted via the criminal justice route either from the courts or prisons. Lee and Warrener (2005) outline the details of the provision under this Part of the Act. Lee *et al.* (2005) provide an insight into the lives of mentally disordered offenders when detained under the Act. The provisions of this Part of the Act empower the court or the Home Secretary to divert mentally ill people who have committed offences or prisoners respectively away from the penal system, in order that these persons can be assessed or treated in hospital. Section 41 or section 49 of this Part of the Act refers to discharge restriction imposed by the court or the Home Secretary respectively; this also implies that leave of absence cannot be granted by the RMO. For persons to whom section 41 applies for the purpose of public protection from serious harm, leave of absence from the detaining hospital can only be granted by the Home Secretary. In relation to prisoners, where section 49 applies, the hospital authority must ensure that the individual is returned to prison when assessment or treatment is completed.

Risk assessment and management are serious considerations for service users detained under Part III of the Act. In general, detained persons where a discharge restriction applies are held in secured hospitals where access and movements are restricted. Staff working with this client group should also be aware of the interface between detention and the criminal justice system. Escorting clients and providing evidence with respect to the individuals' mental health status to the courts may be duties undertaken by staff.

Part IV of the Act provides the legal authority for treatment to be administered under detention. Chapters 15 and 16 of the *Code of Practice* (Department of Health 1999a) provide guidance in respect of consent to treatment. Fennell (1996) provides a critical review of the legal system and historical overview of psychiatric treatment in hospitals In addition, the biennial reports published by the Mental Health Act Commission (MHAC) offer an overview of the operational issues experienced by hospital staff in respect of treatment administered to detained persons. The MHAC also publishes practice guides to supplement the *Code of Practice*.

The provisions under Part IV apply to people detained for treatment, i.e. sections 3 (civil detention), 37 (Part III, admitted via the court) and 47 (Part III, admitted from prison). These are compulsory treatment orders but the routes of admission to hospital are different. Medication may be administered to detained individuals without consent in the first three months of detention, after which period the RMO is obliged to negotiate consent with the service user (Department of Health 1999a). A record of the negotiated consent must be made in the medical records. If the individual refuses to consent, a second opinion must be sought from the MHAC (section 58). Staff involved in the administration of medication must make themselves aware of the date when the individual commenced treatment and when consent is due. They must also be aware of the medication to which an individual has consented. Further, the limit of dosages recommended in the British National Formulary must be adhered to.

This Part IV of the Act regulates rare treatment options such as psycho-surgery (section 57, see Chapter 14 of this book). There is provision to allow emergency treatment for which staff must satisfy themselves that the treatment proposed is immediately necessary to save lives or to prevent serious deterioration of the condition or to alleviate serious sufferings or to prevent dangerous behaviour (Department of Health 1999a). For example, a detainee becomes extremely disturbed and the behaviour represents a risk to the individual or/and others; the RMO may decide to administer medication that provides the immediate effect of preventing serious harm or deterioration in the condition. The treatment given as an emergency must not be 'irreversible or hazardous' (Department of Health 1999a). The controversial treatment electroconvulsive therapy (ECT) may be administered following approval by the second opinion authorised by the MHAC despite refusal by the service user.

There has been much intense debate concerning the potential ethical and moral dilemmas regarding whether an individual should receive treatment in the community in the context of civil liberty. It is a right of mental health service users to refuse treatment, but that right could have disastrous consequences if individuals are not being continuously assessed and closely monitored by mental health services. There had been cases where individuals' behaviour was of great risk to themselves and others, and consequently they committed serious offences. These debates had informed the amendment of the current Act in the Mental Health (Patients in the Community) Act 1995 (Her Majesty's Stationery Office, 1995a), which introduced supervised discharge (section 25A) and the Government's intention to amend the current Act further to introduce supervised treatment in the community.

PROTECTION OF DETAINED PERSONS

The MHAC has the overall function of ensuring that the MHA 1983 is implemented within the legal framework (section 121) and that good practice is in place. Members of MHAC visit hospitals, sometimes unannounced, where there are detained persons and interview detained individuals in private. They may investigate complaints raised by the individuals in respect of their detention.

Detained individuals may apply to the Mental Health Review Tribunal (MHRT) for a review of the detention order. The MHRT has the power to discharge an individual from detention. It is essential that staff inform detained persons of their rights. Currently, hospital managers also have the power to discharge patients; there was an intention to abolish this provision in the proposed reform of the mental health legislation. The specific duties of the hospital managers can be found in the *Code of Practice* (Department of Health 1999a).

Section 117 requires detaining authorities to provide after-care for people who had been detained under the treatment orders (sections 3, 37 and 47) following discharge. After-care services may include assistance with securing appropriate housing and welfare benefits, follow-up care by psychiatric staff to continue to monitor the effects of treatment and mental state. Follow-up care may also involve the provision of ongoing therapeutic interventions. Supervised discharge (section 25A) was introduced under the Mental Health (Patients in the Community) Act 1995 in an attempt to provide a legal framework to care for those vulnerable individuals in the community following discharge from the treatment orders. However, supervised discharge does not include compulsory treatment.

Individuals incapable of managing their affairs such as large sums of money or other assets may be referred to the new Court of Protection, which has been reformed under the Mental Capacity Act 2005 (Her Majesty's Stationery Office 2005). It is an offence under section 127 for staff to ill-treat or neglect persons detained in hospital or in the community, subject to supervised discharge or guardianship. Furthermore, it is also illegal to assist detained persons to leave hospital without leave of absence (section 128). For staff working in secure environments such as special hospitals where the majority of the users are detained under Part III of the Act, the withholding of mail or correspondence under section 134 is subject to review by the MHAC.

The following scenario of John illustrates the different routes of admission under the MHA 1983.

Scenario

John had become mentally unwell for the first time; his GP attempted to treat him but later decided that he required specialist mental health services. A referral was made to the local psychiatric services. John was visited at home by staff from the psychiatric service and it was found that he was very unwell and not willing to accept treatment voluntarily. A further assessment was set up in order that an assessment under the MHA could be carried out (Figures 6.1 and 6.2).

THE GOVERNMENT'S INTENTION TO AMEND THE CURRENT ACT

One of the amendments the Government intends to make to the current Act, which has been subject to intense debate, is replacing the 'treatability test' for the detention of people with a psychopathic disorder or mental impairment; the current Act requires that treatment 'is likely to alleviate or prevent a deterioration' of the condition. There is intention to replace it with 'a test that appropriate treatment must be available' for all individuals detained under compulsory powers (Department of Health 2006). While there is broad consensus that unless appropriate treatment is available compulsory powers should not be used, however the availability of appropriate treatment does not imply that the treatment available is necessary. Hence, applying this criteria to all categories of mental disorder could risk extending the use of compulsory powers. On the other hand, the lack of availability of appropriate treatment could also risk mentally ill people being deprived of treatment There is an urgent need to clarify what constitutes 'appropriate treatment' and whether the Government intends to ensure appropriate treatment is available throughout the country; otherwise the treatment of mentally ill people will join the 'postcode lottery' phenomenon, which could have far-reaching implications. Readers should be aware that the term 'psychopathic disorder' is often used interchangeably with 'personality disorder'.

John is assessed.

Attendance by the GP and a psychiatrist approved under the MHA
is required, and a recommendation for section 2 is made. This was
supported by an ASW, who made an application to the hospital.
The decision made by all had been reached by interviewing John
and his family. The ASW made the necessary arrangements for
admission to hospital.

John is admitted to hospital under section 2 of the MHA1983.

John's right under the MHA is read to him by staff. He may decide
to appeal against his detention to the MHRT or the hospital
managers. The hospital formally informs his nearest relative, as
required by the Act. John is subject to assessment or assessment
followed by treatment. The period of detention does not exceed 28
days. John may be granted leave of absence under section 17. John
may be discharged from detention if he becomes better and willing
to accept treatment informally.

John is refusing treatment and his conditionis deteriorating.

A further assessment under the MHA is made. His GP and the
psychiatrist, who is approved under the Act, made a
recommendation for section 3, which is a treatment order leading
up to 6 months. This was supported by the ASW, who made an
application to the hospital for detention under section 3. If John is
known to the psychiatric service as a service user, the staff may
decide that he be detained under section 3 without having to use a
formal assessment order, which is section 2.

John is now detained under section 3 of the MHA.

As John's MHA status has changed, the staff are required to read to
him his rights under section 3, and the hospital has to inform his
nearest relative formally as required by the Act. John may be
interviewed by the MHAC if they were visiting or he could write to
them to investigate any complaint he may have in respect of his
detention. John is obliged to accept treatment. John is subject to
Part IV of the Act if his treatment proceeds beyond 12 weeks, at
which time his RMO is required to seek his consent to continue
treatment. If John refuses, a second opinion is sought from the
MHAC in order that he may be treated compulsorily.

John gets better.

The multidisciplinary team may decide that John should be allowed
leave of absence, and the RMO authorises section 17. The team
begins to negotiate with John and his family about discharge and
after-care arrangements under section 117.

Discharge is arranged with aftercare arranged.

Figure 6.1 Assessment and treatment under the MHA

The convicted person is in prison, but becomes mentally unwell. The person may then be transferred to hospital for treatment under section 47, based on two medical reports.

Applying the same requirements as above, remand prisoners may be sent to hospital under section 48.

Section 49, a restrictive order, is imposed at the same time as sections 47 or 48 as the individuals may not be transferred elsewhere or discharged due to their prisoner status.

Based on the evidence from two medical reports that the individual is mentally ill and requires treatment, the court may decide to send a convicted individual to hospital for treatment under section 37 of the MHA; instead of imposing a prison sentence because of the severity of the offence, Section 41, which is a restriction order, may also be imposed where only the Secretary of State may grant leave of absence. When detained under section 37, the person has similar rights as in section 3.

An interim order, section 38, may be imposed on a convicted individual to be admitted to hospital for the purpose of evaluating his/her mental condition in hospital before a hospital treatment order is made.

Section 35 empowers the court to remand the accused to hospital for the purpose of preparing a medical report on his/her mental condition.
The court may remand the accused under section 36 to hospital for treatment.

Figure 6.2 Alternative routes to admissions under detention for offenders

One of the Government's intentions in the amendment of the current Act is to introduce a form of supervised treatment in the community. This could potentially benefit mentally disordered people being supported and treated within their home environment, enabling them to comply with their treatment plans and facilitating early intervention before reaching crisis level. Supervised treatment in the community could also facilitate early discharge from hospital; reducing the risk of social exclusion, which is often associated with long periods of detention in hospital. There is evidence that the current provision of supervised discharge (section 25A) has resulted in increased community survival rates (Franklin *et al.* 2000). However, the notion of supervised treatment in one's own home is controversial, as being supervised implies an element of compulsion, although the term does not suggest compulsory treatment in the community. There is a risk that civil liberty could be compromised.

THE DISABILITY DISCRIMINATION ACT (DDA) 1995

The DDA (Her Majesty's Stationery Office 1995b) was introduced in 1996 and aims to end discrimination faced by people who are disabled. DDA 1995 covers the following areas:

- access to goods and services
- buying or renting land or property
- employment.

Under the DDA 1995:

- it becomes unlawful to treat disabled people less favourably than other people for a reason related to their disability
- employers have to make reasonable adjustments to provide extra help or make changes for disabled people
- physical features to overcome physical barriers for access to premises must be made.

Disability is defined as 'a physical or mental impairment which has a substantial and long term adverse effect on a person's ability to carry out normal day to day activities' (Minister for Disabled People 1996). The term 'mental impairment' relates to people who have a learning disability and to those who have a mental illness (Minister for Disabled People 1996). Guidance as to what constitutes 'substantial and long term' and 'normal day to day activities' are provided by the Minister for Disabled People (1996).

It is important that staff working in all care environments, and in particular those working within the sphere of mental health, familiarise themselves with the implications of working practices as a result of the DDA 1995. For example, if a mental health service user is unable to participate in activities as a result of any lack of a suitable aid, or when staff organise activities that did not include people who have problems in participating as a result of their disability, staff in these situations should consider if reasonable adjustments could be made to enable the individuals to participate. In any case, it is good practice to adopt an anti-discrimination stance at all times. It is illegal not to employ a person who suffers from a serious and enduring mental health problem on the grounds of the illness. Staff should support and advocate on behalf of long-term mental health service users in seeking employment and work towards an agenda of social inclusion.

The Disability Rights Commission (DRC) was formed in 2000 by Act of Parliament. Its function is to eliminate discrimination faced by disabled people and promote equality of opportunity. The organisation offers services such as a helpline, conciliation service, advice and information. There is a casework team that will research and investigate potential cases of discrimination.

THE HUMAN RIGHTS ACT (HRA) 1998

The HRA 1998 (Her Majesty's Stationery Office 1998) incorporates the rights of the European Convention on Human Rights (ECHR) and has been in force in England since 2000. The HRA aims: 'to protect the human rights of individuals against the abuse of power by the State, meaning any public authority' (Daw 2000). The health service, as a public authority, has a duty to exercise its powers in a way that is compatible with the ECHR. This duty is reflected in the first guiding principle enshrined in the *Code of Practice* (Department of Health 1999a);

it stipulates: 'recognition of basic human rights under the European Convention on Human Rights'.

Human rights have been applied to challenge mental health practice on numerous occasions in the courts. The following Articles highlight the relationship of human rights with mental health practice:

ARTICLE 2: THE RIGHT TO LIFE

This Article requires hospitals, which represent public bodies, to have in place policies that protect patients' lives and a system by which accidents or untoward incidents are investigated. For mental health staff, issues such as the use of force and the level of force used when restraining violent and absconding patients are pertinent. The MHAC (2003) cited the death of David Bennett and the unlawful killing of Roger Sylvester, both mental health service users, as results of the application of control and restraint techniques. The training provided in the use of restraint is crucial to achieving a level of awareness and practice that is compatible with the requirements of the human rights of patients (Home Office 2000).

ARTICLE 3: FREEDOM FROM TORTURE OR INHUMAN OR DEGRADING TREATMENT

A Broadmoor patient (*A* v. *UK* [1980] 3 EHRR, 131; cited in Eldergill 2000) took his complaint to the ECHR. It was alleged that the seclusion room where he was detained amounted to inhumane conditions, that he was deprived of clothing, adequate furnishing and that the room had been unsanitary, inadequately lit and ventilated. A settlement was reached with the Government in that compensation was paid to the patient. It could be suggested as a result of this case that, while caring for patients with challenging behaviour is not an easy task, staff have a duty to ensure that the conditions in which service users are cared for are not inhumane.

Inhumane treatment may include (Home Office 2000):

- serious physical assaults
- inhuman detention conditions or restraints
- failing to provide or withdrawing proper medical help to a person with a serious illness
- a threat of torture, if it is real and immediate.

In the case of *Herczegfalvy* v. *Austria* (1992) 15 EHRR 437, the client complained that he was administered food and psychotropic drugs forcibly and was isolated and handcuffed to a security bed for several weeks. While his extreme aggression and violence justified the use of coercive measures and his deteriorating physical and mental condition warranted treatment in the form of food and medication, the ECHR determined that, as a general rule, a therapeutic necessity cannot be regarded as inhumane or degrading but the length of time in which the handcuffs and security bed were used appeared worrying (Eldergill 2000). The key issue was that any form of treatment should be subject to regular review and the least restrictive alternative measure must be initiated. Therefore, practice must be consistent with the guiding principle in the *Code of Practice*:

> be given any necessary treatment or care in the least controlled and segregated facilities compatible with ensuring their own health or safety or the safety of other people. (Department of Health 1999a).

The MHAC (2003) cited the cases of *Munjaz* v. *Mersey Care NHS Trust* and *S.* v. *Airedale NHS Trust* involving the use of seclusion in mental health facilities; the users sought legal challenges applying human rights legislation. It was made clear that improper use of seclusion and without due regard to the users' welfare could violate Article 3. The MHAC (2003) reiterated that compliance with the guidance provided by the *Code of Practice* (Department of Health 1999a) was essential.

ARTICLE 5: PERSONAL FREEDOM

The process leading to the compulsory detention of individuals must have its basis in law, and therefore those mental health professionals accepting detained patients on behalf of the authority must have training and sound knowledge in the application of the mental health legislation in order that they can fulfil their duty properly and within the confines of the law. Staff must also be aware of the guiding principle in the *Code of Practice*, that individuals should:

> be discharged from detention or other powers provided by the Act as soon as it is clear that their application is no longer justified. (Department of Health 1999a).

Continued detention without satisfying the legal criteria may be in breach of Article 5. Hence, regular review and bringing attention to others, of the user's mental state is a crucial duty of the staff.

Other rights under Article 5 that apply to service users in mental health care are that they should:

- be informed in language that they understand
- be able to challenge the lawfulness of detention before an independent judicial body, and that they have the right to be released and obtain compensation
- have detention reviewed at (various) intervals.

The reading of rights to detained persons is an example of this obligation, which requires rights to be read/given in an appropriate language by mental health practitioners. There have been several cases where detained persons have challenged the legality of their detention and the time it had taken the MHRT to review their cases, in the courts under Article 5 of the HRA.

The Bournewood (*R* v. *Bournewood Community and Mental Health Trust*) case highlighted the lack of clarity in law relating to persons who do not have the mental capacity to consent and yet are not allowed to leave by staff. It involved a man with a learning disability who was living in the community but who had been admitted to hospital as a result of disturbed behaviour at a day centre. He was incapable of consenting to admission and was not allowed to leave hospital, despite that he was not detained there. His carers were not allowed to visit, and they subsequently challenged the legality of his admission in court. The House of Lords ruled that, based on the common law doctrine of necessity, treatment could be provided to persons who are incapable of consenting when it was in the best interest of the individuals. However, Daw (2000) suggests that common law is unlikely to satisfy detention under Article 5. This scenario can be reflected in facilities that care for people who are mentally confused or have a learning disability. Staff working with this client group should be aware of individuals who are not allowed to leave and yet do not have the capacity to give consent to remain in hospital or care facility, or receive treatment.

ARTICLE 6: RIGHT TO A FAIR TRIAL

For persons detained in mental health facilities, this refers to the right of having a fair hearing at an MHRT. Some may require the services of an interpreter in order that they fully understand the proceedings of the hearing. Staff have a duty to ensure that independent interpreters who speak the appropriate languages are available for MHRT hearings.

ARTICLE 8: PRIVATE LIFE AND FAMILY

It includes the:

- right to respect for your private and family life
- right to live your life with privacy as is reasonable in a democratic society, taking into account the rights and freedoms of others
- right to have information about you kept private and confidential
- freedom to choose your sexual identity
- freedom to choose how you look and dress
- freedom from intrusion by the media.

This includes the right of mental health service users to have sexual relationships. Practice areas must have guidance for staff to act appropriately in order to respect the right of service users to develop sexual relationships. Staff should be aware of issues concerning cultural differences, gender issues and differences in sexual orientation of the users.

Personal searches on wards, the interception of mail in high-security hospitals, not allowing family members to visit patients and taking blood samples may arguably be in breach of Article 8 unless the grounds for this can be justified as above. The measures taken must be proportional to what is necessary.

The right to private life also includes information such as clinical records being kept private and confidential. The giving of information to relatives or others requires careful consideration as disclosure could arguably be interpreted as a violation of this right. The objection of the patient should not be treated lightly in circumstances such as: information given to the nearest relative under section 133 of the Mental Health Act 1983, invitation to family members to participate in a Care Programme Approach or after-care planning meetings.

ARTICLE 9: FREEDOM OF BELIEF

In mental health care, this includes having arrangements for religious practice in place and to be flexible with working practices and having a protocol with the user and family as to what is acceptable practice and what is not in order to enable staff to support service users in their practising their faith or religious beliefs.

ARTICLE 10: FREE EXPRESSION

Article 10 may be relevant to those who 'whistleblow' on aspects of poor care and illegal detention; staff may compromise the welfare of service users or others under Articles 2, 3 and 5 if they do not exercise the freedom to express their views for the protection of service users.

ARTICLE 11: FREE ASSEMBLY AND ASSOCIATION

Restriction of a user's right to go where he/she pleases and to associate with whom he/she pleases is a contravention of Article 11. The curtailment of a mental health user's freedom of movement must be based on a sound assessment of the potential danger that the patient or others may be in. Restrictions must be justified by reference to special reasons and legal tests.

ARTICLE 12: MARRIAGE

This is an absolute right that can only be curtailed in specific circumstances; most of these will relate to instances where consent is questionable. The mentally disordered offender who is detained in a special hospital (for example Rampton, Broadmoor or Ashworth) is allowed to marry while resident in the institution; however, as with ordinary prisoners, they may not be allowed to consummate the marriage. This position may be challenged in the future as a curtailment of Article 8 (the right to family life).

ARTICLE 14: FREEDOM FROM DISCRIMINATION

Discrimination means treating people in similar situations differently, or those in different situations in the same way, without proper justification. Examples of the grounds of discrimination that the ECHR prohibits (Home Office 2000) are:

- sex
- race
- colour
- language
- religion
- political or other opinion
- national or social origin
- association with a national minority
- property
- birth or other status.

The ECHR also protects individuals from discrimination on other grounds of:

- sexual orientation
- whether they are born inside or outside a marriage
- disability
- marital status
- age.

A common example of discrimination takes the form of rehabilitation activities in which men and women are expected to participate together. Some cultures advocate the segregation of the sexes except where a formal union has taken place. When women or men refuse to participate, no alternative is offered or the individuals are seen as being uncooperative in their treatment plan, this could be interpreted as discrimination.

It is well documented that black patients feel that they are being discriminated against by mental health services (Sainsbury Centre for Mental Health 1998) and that this group of users are detained more than their white counterparts (Department of Health 1999b). These differences could be seen as discrimination on the grounds of race, colour and sex. The second guiding principle in the *Code of Practice* (Department of Health 1999a) reflects the requirements set out in Articles 8, 9 and 14.

THE MENTAL INCAPACITY ACT (MIA) 2005

The MIA 2005 will come into force in April 2007. It provides a 'statutory framework to empower and protect vulnerable people who are not able to make their own decision' (Department for Constitutional Affairs 2006). A code of practice will be published to guide professionals in their implementation of the Act, and it will be a duty of care for staff to follow the code.

Staff working with people with memory loss, severe learning disability or anyone who is mentally incapacitated albeit temporarily should be aware of their duties under the Act. The Act sets out a decision-specific test for 'assessing whether a person lacks capacity to take a particular decision at a particular time' (Department for Constitutional Affairs 2006). The Act is underpinned by five key principles:

1. a presumption that everyone can make their own decisions
2. individuals have the right to be supported to make their own decisions
3. individuals have the right to make decisions that appear unwise or bad
4. when a decision is made for someone who lacks capacity, it must be in their best interests
5. any action taken on behalf of someone who lacks capacity must be the least restrictive of their basic rights and freedom.

The Act sets out rules for persons giving care or treatment to individuals who are incapacitated and that 'the best interests checklist' is followed to enable a care giver to decide what is in the best interest of the incapacitated person. Under the Act, there are clear rules with safeguards in respect of advanced decisions to refuse treatment. An advanced decision is a decision made by individuals in respect of their refusal to receive treatment if they lose incapacity in the future (Department for Constitutional Affairs 2006). Individuals may appoint lasting powers of attorney (LPA) to act on their behalf if they lose capacity in the future.

The new Court of Protection may appoint a deputy to act in the best interests of an individual if there was no LPA appointed. A new body called the Public Guardian will be the registering authority for LPAs and deputies. There is provision for an independent mental capacity advocate, who makes representations about the incapacitated person's wishes or feelings, for example highlighting factors that are relevant to the decision-makers.

The MIA 2005 lays down strict rules about research involving people who do not have capacity to consent. Staff should make themselves familiar with the rules if conducting research using this client group as a sample.

CONCLUSION

This chapter has provided some insight into how various aspects of legislation may impact on everyone's lives at different times depending on the circumstances. Professionals should be aware of an individual's situation when caring for people within the legal frameworks and adopt good practice at all times. Frequently in mental health work, one or more aspects of the law may affect individuals at the same time. Some mental health service users are particularly vulnerable when unwell; it is the practitioner's duty to uphold their rights under different legislation.

REFERENCES

Daw R (2000) *The impact of the Human Rights Act on Disabled People*. London, Disability Rights Commission.

Department of Constitutional Affairs (2006) Mental Capacity Act, http://www.dca.gov.uk/menincap/legis.htm, accessed 20 July 2006.

Department of Health (1999a) *Code of Practice Mental Health Act 1983*. London, The Stationery Office.

Department of Health (1999b) *A System Review of Research Relating to the Mental Health Act 1983*. London, The Stationery Office.

Department of Health (2006) Mental Health Bill: Written Ministerial Statement, http://www.dh.gov.uk/PolicyAndGuidance/HealthAndSocialCareTopics/MentalHealth/MentalHealth Article/fs/en?CONTENT_ID=4132141&chk=bAKou7, accessed 7 July 2006.

Eldergill A (2000) *Human Rights Act 1998 & Mental Health. Paper to Department of Health*. London, Department of Health.

Fennell P (1996) *Treatment Without Consent*. London, Routledge.

Franklin D, Pinfold V, Bindman J, Thornicroft G (2000) Consultant psychiatrists' experiences of using supervised discharge. *Psychiatric Bulletin* **24**: 412–415.

Home Office (2000) *Study Guide Human Rights Act 1998*. London, Home Office.

Her Majesty's Stationery Office (1995a) Mental Health (Patients in the Community) Act 1995, http://www.opsi.gov.uk/ACTS/acts1995/Ukpga_19950052_ en_1.htm, accessed 6 July 2006.

Her Majesty's Stationery Office (1995b) The Disability Discrimination Act 1995, http://www.opsi.gov.uk/acts/acts1995/1995050.htm, accessed 6 July 2006.

Her Majesty's Stationery Office (1998) The Human Rights Act 1998, http://www.opsi.gov.uk/ACTS/acts1998/19980042.htm, accessed 6 July 2006.

Her Majesty's Stationery Office (2005) Mental Capacity Act 2005, http://www.opsi.gov.uk/acts/acts2005/20050009.htm, accessed 6 July 2006.

Jones R (2004) *Mental Health Act Manual*. London, Sweet & Maxwell.

Lee S, Warrener J (2005) Chapter 4. In Littlechild B, Fearns D (eds), *Mental Disorder and Criminal Justice*. Lyme Regis, Russell House.

Lee S, Warrener J, Cloudsdale S (2005) Chapter 5. In Littlechild B, Fearns D (eds), *Mental Disorder and Criminal Justice*. Lyme Regis, Russell House.

Mental Health Act Commission (2003) *Tenth Biennial Report*. London, The Stationery Office.

Minister for Disabled People (1996) *The Disability Discrimination Act – Definition of Disability: DL 60 From October 1996*. London, The Stationery Office.

Sainsbury Centre for Mental Health (1998) *Keys to engagement*. London, Sainsbury Centre for Mental Health.

7 Anxiety Disorders

T. BEARY

INTRODUCTION

This chapter aims to describe how anxiety, while being essential to everyday functioning, can be detrimental to the person's welfare if not properly controlled. It will focus on the treatments that are utilised to care for people when anxiety becomes a disorder.

Anxiety is a general human feeling – its representation and how it is dealt with is exclusive to each person. The degree of anxiety that a person suffers depends upon their own reaction and length of exposure to a situation or object that has the capacity to cause that person stress (Davies & Armstrong 2002). It is also usually proportional to the perceived threat to the person and it can prompt the body to react in an appropriate manner in order to maintain the person's safety and welfare. Once the perceived threat is removed or dealt with, the level of anxiety usually subsides. Anxiety can be mild, moderate or severe in its presentation. It can also have a physical, psychological, social or emotional impact on the person. According to Thomas (2004) 'anxiety becomes a disorder when it is consistent, intense and debilitating, to the extent that it disrupts your life'.

Everybody will experience some anxiety in their life, and this is a typical reaction to certain matters which the person perceives as stressful at that particular time. Reflect on the way a person may feel when having to undertake an examination. Their palms probably feel clammy; the person might feel unsettled and restless with thoughts and feelings preoccupying their brain. Unconsciously, their heart is beating faster than normal in line with their increased breathing, but perhaps they do not notice this at the time. Imagine a person having to stand in front of their classmates to read aloud or do a presentation for the first time. They almost certainly are conscious of the fact that they are standing alone in front of their friends and their teacher. They are probably more conscious of the fact that their mouth is dry and, despite their best efforts, their words are muddled and it is somewhat difficult for them to speak clearly. However, once the task has been completed (finishing the examination, concluding the reading or presentation), all of the aforementioned symptoms later subside, with or without the person noticing that this has happened. This is the body's reaction to stressful situations and experiences of restlessness

Caring for Adults with Mental Health Problems   Edited by I. Peate and S. Chelvanayagam
© 2006 John Wiley & Sons, Ltd

towards some object or situation. Healy (2005) classes this as 'stage fright', and it can occur when people are placed in situations that require unfamiliar functioning in front of others. It is similar to a defence mechanism that generally allows us as human beings to survive and to effectively deal with situations. As a defence mechanism, it can be viewed as a positive feeling since it warns people of potential dangers and can spur them on to react appropriately. This is usually referred to as the 'fight or flight' response and, therefore, is present in each and every one of us.

Semple *et al.* define anxiety as:

> a normal and adaptive response to stress and danger which is pathological if prolonged, severe, or out of keeping with the real threat of the external situation (Semple *et al.* 2005)

Feelings of anxiety do not pose a problem if the body reacts to a situation or danger appropriately in order to protect the person in question. It is estimated that between 8% and 12% of people experience a persistent level of anxiety in their lifetime (Muir-Cochrane 2003). However, these people still function on a daily basis. On the other hand, severe anxiety can lead to an inability to function, which may interfere with the person's overall ability to perform even the simplest of everyday tasks. Muir-Cochrane also states that between 2% and 4% of the population will experience an anxiety disorder that will interfere significantly with their everyday lives. Problems occur when the level of reaction to the situation or object is so great that it begins to obstruct the person's welfare and hinders their ability to lead a full and active life. The person may display behaviours that are not in keeping with their character, which could be perceived as an inability to cope with life's situations. In addition, it must be recognised that, while it may be devastating, severe anxiety also has the potential to be life-threatening.

Scenario One: Anxiety

Mary, a 37-year-old secretary, is single and lives alone. She usually has a good network of friends within and outside the workplace. Recently, while on a shopping trip in the town, Mary was attacked and thrown to the ground, during which she sustained bruising to her face and a fracture to her wrist. Her handbag was also snatched during this attack, which contained, amongst other things, her house keys. Consequently, Mary now feels frightened to leave the house and any attempts to encourage Mary to do so are met with great resistance. She is currently on sick leave from her job and now relies on her friends to do her shopping. Within the past week, Mary has called the police to the house in the early hours of the morning on three separate occasions. She is unable to sleep at night and believes that she can hear somebody trying to use her stolen keys to gain entry to her home. On the third occasion, while the police were at the house, Mary suddenly collapsed and her heart stopped beating.

> She was taken to the local hospital, where she was successfully treated. While in hospital, she was referred to and seen by a psychiatrist, who is currently treating Mary for anxiety.

PHYSIOLOGY ASSOCIATED WITH ANXIETY

Fundamental to understanding anxiety and how it affects the person are the endocrine and nervous systems in the body. These are the body's main regulatory systems – the nervous system relays impulses to and from the brain via sensory receptors; the endocrine system governs the pituitary gland, which is linked to the hypothalamus in the brain. The hypothalamus also functions as a centre that combines hormonal and autonomic nervous activity (Van Wynsberghe *et al.* 1995).

The nervous system is essential for functioning as it is responsible for delivering messages from different parts of the body to the brain via the spinal cord, and vice versa. Trickett (1996) compares the nervous system to that of a 'network of communication between various parts of the body, rather like a telephone exchange'. Therefore, it is essential that all aspects of the system are operating correctly. The nervous system comprises two main components – the central nervous system and the autonomic nervous system.

THE CENTRAL NERVOUS SYSTEM

The central nervous system is composed of the brain and spinal cord. It is responsible for receiving and understanding all stimuli and assisting the body in reacting accordingly. The central nervous system is also involved in fine movement and coordination. Essential to the central nervous system are cells called neurons that have the ability to respond to stimuli (excitability) and to transmit a signal (conductivity) (Van Wynsberghe *et al.* 1995).

THE AUTONOMIC NERVOUS SYSTEM

This part of the nervous system comprises two parts – the sympathetic nervous system and the parasympathetic nervous system. Both systems work in harmony with each other, and it is this balance of working that is essential to the stability of mind and body. It allows people to make decisions in certain situations and act in direct proportion to the perceived threat.

The sympathetic nervous system works when the person is faced with a problem or situation that needs consideration. The response of the sympathetic nervous system is to release hormones called adrenaline (or epinephrine), noradrenaline and cortisol from the adrenal glands. The request for this is a direct response from the hypothalamus and pituitary gland via the sympathetic nervous system. The level of released hormones is usually proportional to the perceived problem or situation at

Physical symptoms	Cognitive symptoms
Heart beating faster	Increased alertness
Palpitations	Difficulty in concentrating
Feeling faint	Distraction
Rapid breathing	Thoughts are unclear
Dry mouth	Confusion
Lump in throat	Fear of losing control
Rigidity of muscles in limbs	Increased awareness
Nausea/vomiting	Fearful ideation present
Dilation of pupils	Increased vigilance
Feeling of wanting to urinate	
Sweaty palms	
Behavioural symptoms	**Emotional symptoms**
Restlessness	Fear of the unknown
Fidgeting	Poor self-worth
Fight or flight	Crying
Immobility	Possible lack of support
Stammering when talking	Screaming
Reduced co-ordination	Feeling depressed

Figure 7.1 Changes associated with anxiety

that time. As a result of this release, heart and breathing rates increase, pupils dilate and salivary and sweat glands are activated (Figure 7.1). This supports the fright, fight or flight responses as the body is at a sensitive state of eagerness to appropriately deal with the perceived problem or situation. Anxiety levels are increased at this time. This increased anxiety within the person prepares them for an appropriate course of action in order to deal effectively with the situation. All energy at this time is directed towards the activity.

Once the situation has been dealt with and the person can relax, the parasympathetic system comes into play. All of the aforementioned physiological changes are reversed and a balance is promoted within the body that allows it to relax and replenish itself in readiness for the next situation. Levels of anxiety decrease, and this allows the person to reflect on the encounter. It is possible that personal learning is achieved in the process. This learned information may be stored and could assist the person in the future with similar situations.

The balance between the sympathetic and the parasympathetic systems is essential to the welfare of the person. Mild or moderate levels of anxiety can act as a driving force that may increase productivity and performance while maintaining the body's ability to function. It is also accepted that the sympathetic nervous system tends to be more dominant than the parasympathetic system, taking into account the stresses of living. The parasympathetic system must come into play at some stage to promote a balance within the body. However, problems present when this balance is not synchronised and the body is not given adequate time to relax and replenish itself in preparation for the next demanding event. Coupled to anxiety are the problems associated with stress. This occurs when there is a prolonged and constant exposure to situations, which could result in mental and physical exhaustion.

STRESS

Stress is 'a specific kind of biological reaction, which can be expressed emotionally' (Barker 1993). Problems occur when exposure to stress is extended over an interval of time and when that stress is allowed to attain excessive levels. This can weaken the person's capacity to cope with their everyday problems and, in turn, could lead to a breakdown in the mental health of the person in question. However, to avoid this situation, it is essential that the sources of the stress are identified and modified accordingly. There are three stages to the stress response (Seyle 1956):

1. Alarm: reaction to the situation
2. Resistance: continued reaction, resulting in prolonged release of cortisol
3. Exhaustion: inability to cope, requires intervention.

Problems with stress begin to occur when continued reaction is prolonged over a period of time. While cortisol is one of the body's essential hormones, too much cortisol in the system can have detrimental effects. Cortisol is responsible for inhibiting infection, especially viral infection. It is also responsible for converting carbohydrates to glucose to give the body energy. However, if the level of cortisol is sustained at a high level in the body, it can interfere with the body's other internal mechanisms, especially those which promote the ability to rest and sleep. Consequently, this results in increased overactivity and does not allow the body time to refresh itself. The person is more susceptible to infections and may develop depression due to a changing level of neurotransmitters in the brain. With the sympathetic nervous system continuously working overtime, energy levels will be depleted when the body is reliant on energy stores in times of true crisis.

CLASSIFICATION OF ANXIETY DISORDERS

Muir-Cochrane (2003) suggests that the most common anxiety problems are classified as follows:

- generalised anxiety disorder
- phobias
- obsessive-compulsive disorder
- post-traumatic stress
- panic disorder.

However, Muir-Cochrane (2003) states that 'anxiety is one of the most common treatable mental disorders'. Anxiety can also be present in some other mental disorders such as depression; high levels of anxiety can trigger suicidal thoughts (Trickett 1996). Semple *et al.* (2005) class this as 'differential diagnosis' – it can occur as a part of another disorder. Therefore, it is essential that anxiety disorders are taken into consideration and treated appropriately. If not, anxiety could exacerbate an already established mental disorder and give rise to undue distress to the person.

GENERALISED ANXIETY DISORDER

Generalised anxiety disorder (GAD) results in 27% of people being referred to a psychiatrist for consultation by their general practitioner (GP) (Katona & Robertson 2000). Eight per cent of patients seen in the psychiatric out-patient clinic will present with GAD. It is more prevalent in females than males. GAD can be acute or chronic, the latter being prevalent for a period of six months or more. It is sometimes known as 'free-floating anxiety'. GAD could also have its basis in childhood – issues such as separation in childhood which have not been resolved fully and are subsequently carried over into adulthood.

One way to describe GAD is that of excessive worrying, with or without a cause. The person may experience excessive and persistent feelings of apprehension about a number of everyday issues such as work performance and family matters (Smith 2000). These persistent feelings may or may not be well founded but to the sufferer feel very real. Furthermore, the excessive worrying is invasive and begins to spill over into the person's life. The person may appear nervous and on edge, may not seem to relax and the ability to easily startle them is also evident. Restless behaviour (for example tapping of the feet, moving about in a chair, looking around in anticipation of something happening) and sleeping difficulties may be reported. There may be other sources of worry that may only serve to compound the problem. The autonomic nervous system at this time is active with possible evidence of an increase in heart rate, dilated pupils and an increase in respiratory rate. In some situations, the person may report that the heart is beating so loudly that others can hear it. Walking and maintaining balance can be difficult at this time because of muscle rigidity or tremor.

PHOBIAS

A phobia can be defined as 'a pathologically strong fear of a particular event or thing' (Martin 2003). In relation to phobias, the person experiences extremes of fear, but sometimes there are no specific reasons for this. The behaviour of the person is usually out of proportion to the stimulus that causes the anxiety. The person focuses on the situation and genuinely believes that they are going to come to some harm. Attempts at reassuring the person can be difficult. This can affect the person so much that they tend to completely avoid the situation or stimulus which provokes these feelings within them. It is also claimed that avoidance of the situation could be a part of the problem when coming to terms or effectively dealing with the phobia (Spielberger 1987).

Phobias can be divided into three categories (Puri 2000):

1. specific phobia
2. social phobia
3. agoraphobia.

Specific phobia

About 17% of people seen by psychiatrists will have a specific phobia, and the ratio for this is equal between males and females (Katona & Robertson 2000). Conversely, Puri (2000) argues that it is more prevalent in the female population and suggests that phobias usually commence either in childhood or early adult life and, if left untreated, the person may experience years of anguish. Specific phobia is precise and the person is explicit in relation to their fear and, sometimes, as to how they will react when faced with this. A specific phobia can be wide and varied and can range from, for example, fear of animals (both wild and/or domesticated), flying, heights, darkness to fear of enclosed spaces. In addition, the person can exhibit signs and symptoms of their phobia, even if they only anticipate an encounter with this. However, if the person is faced with their phobia, it can lead to immense fear and dread. Some people become so disturbed by this ordeal that it may lead to panic.

Scenario Two: Specific phobia

Oliver is 27 and works as a car mechanic. When Oliver was eight years old, he was playing football with his cousin in the back garden when the football accidentally went into the next-door-neighbour's garden. Oliver climbed over the fence to retrieve the football, but when he was climbing over the fence he was attacked by the neighbour's dog. The dog pulled Oliver off the fence. Oliver sustained severe injuries to his face, neck and hands, which required surgery and prolonged hospitalisation. Since this episode, Oliver cannot look at or stroke a dog of any breed. If a dog comes close to Oliver, Oliver will freeze and will be unable to move until the animal is removed. When walking down the street, Oliver will purposely cross to the other side of the road if he sees a dog walking towards him, even if this dog is a guide dog with its owner and the dog is on a lead.

Social phobia

A social phobia is an anxiety-provoking reaction that occurs when a person thinks about meeting with others in public. It revolves around the person's fear of being looked at by other people and generally relates to small gatherings as opposed to crowds (Puri 2000). The person can feel that others are watching their every move, thinking that people may be judging their social skills – that is talking in public, eating, drinking – even though this may not be the case. The person may also feel that they will be rejected if they act out of place. As a result, the person isolates themselves from the public and situations that could be perceived as awkward. Social phobia often manifests itself in adolescence and occurs in males and females equally (Puri 2000). It could also result in the person avoiding situations and meetings with members of the opposite sex, probably due to feelings of inadequacy.

If this phobia is left untreated, it could lead to a chronic condition resulting in increased anxiety and social exclusion for the person in question.

Agoraphobia

The word 'agoraphobia' is derived from the Greek *agora*, meaning a marketplace and *phobos*, meaning fear. Despite the popular notion that agoraphobia is a fear of open spaces, Ash asserts that this is not the case and defines agoraphobia as 'a fear of being in public places' (Ash 1997). Consequently, the person avoids public places such as buses, trains, shopping centres or any public place where their level of anxiety could reach such a degree that they would not be able to control this. Agoraphobia is more prevalent in the female population; females account for 66% of sufferers (Katona & Robertson 2000). The onset of agoraphobia can occur at any time from mid to late teens and onwards. If left untreated, the person can spend months, and sometimes years, indoors without going into public places. Agoraphobia can also be known as 'phobic anxiety'.

Scenario Three: Agoraphobia

Paula is an 18-year-old student nurse who recently left home in the countryside to study in London. Paula was very happy to study in London as this was her first time away from home and her first time living in London. Additionally, her training in London could help her career prospects. One weekend, Paula decided to walk into the West End to see the sights of the city. However, when walking on Regent Street, Paula became overwhelmed with the amount of people who were walking towards her. She felt totally bombarded by the crowds of people because she was not used to this. However, this seemed to be repeated everywhere she went, be it on public transportation or in shops. Consequently, Paula avoided crowds and public places and failed to attend her lectures and placements. As a result, her nurse training was terminated. Paula felt envious of her colleagues who appeared to adapt to the way of life in a big city.

OBSESSIVE-COMPULSIVE DISORDER

Obsessive-compulsive disorder (OCD) is defined as 'a chronic and common condition often associated with marked anxiety and depression characterised by obsessions and compulsions' (Semple *et al.* 2005). The obsession relates to thoughts that are constant and disturbing to the person and the compulsion is a driving force that reinforces the idea to act out a certain behaviour, regardless of the effectiveness of this behaviour (Shives & Isaacs 2002). It affects males and females equally and can start in childhood or early adult life. These obsessions and compulsions are usually accompanied with thoughts of distress as the person is fearful of the misfortune or any other associated adversity that could occur if a specific pattern of behaviour is not followed. A typical example of such behaviour is that of repeated hand washing and the danger of contamination. The obsession can lead to the person repeating certain behaviours as a relief to prevent any misfortune, such as contamination, happening. Sadly, such relief is short-lived and the person's anxiety level causes the person to wash their hands repeatedly. In time, the person may develop a ritual for their behaviour that may extend to and interfere with other aspects of their life. When carrying out the ritual, if the person is disturbed, makes a mistake or does not carry out the ritual in a set way, it may result in the procedure having to be started all over again. This reassures the person that the ritual has been carried out appropriately. This could result in the obsession interfering with other essential elements of the person's life. If the level of anxiety in obsessive-compulsive disorder is great, it could lead to further associated psychiatric disorders, such as depression, eating disorders (owing to fear of contamination), alcohol or drug-related problems.

Scenario Four: Obsessive-compulsive disorder

Harry is a 20-year-old man who is a trainee hairdresser in the local town. He has always loved his job and is enthusiastic and eager to learn. Harry's obsessive-compulsive trait started when a lady arrived at the salon one day to have her hair styled. On examining the scalp with his bare hands, Harry noted that the lady had some lesions in her scalp that were oozing. This frightened Harry as he feared that these lesions were contagious. Harry washed his hands but was not convinced that he had done this properly. Following this episode, Harry began to wash his hands on a regular basis, even after touching the equipment in the salon that his colleagues were using. This obsession spilled over into his home life and he began to develop a certain ritual, which he followed religiously. He started to shower or bathe about three times a day. He started getting up earlier each day so that this ritual could be followed. If Harry did not follow his ritual specifically, he would need to start the ritual again from the beginning. Harry's exemplary work attendance began to fade and at times he could not even leave the house because of his obsession. Harry needed to be admitted to a psychiatric unit for treatment.

POST-TRAUMATIC STRESS DISORDER

Post-traumatic stress disorder (PTSD) is an extreme reaction to witnessing or experiencing a traumatic event in a person's life and can happen to anybody. The American Psychiatric Association's (1994) definition of a traumatic event, as cited in Lovell and Richards, suggests that two major issues are present:

first, that the events involved actual or threatened death or serious injury, or a threat to the physical integrity of others; secondly, the person's response involved intense fear, helplessness, or horror (Lovell & Richards 1997).

Examples of situations that could provoke PTSD include torture, war, rape, explosions, crashes and personal physical attacks. Bullying may be added to this list (Thomas 2004). Usually, the person begins to experience flashbacks that can be vivid in nature, as if the person is reliving the experience all over again. This can be characterised by a heightened sense of awareness; the person is overvigilant of everything. There may be an increased startle reaction and the person appears to be ready for any threatening situation. Nightmares of varying degrees related to the event are common, as is insomnia. The person will try to avoid anything that will remind them of the trauma. Personality changes can be evident with the person displaying aloofness, and they may not socialise with others, preferring instead to keep their own company. The ability to create and maintain relationships with members of either sex may be hindered. The person may display feelings of anger or guilt, or they may be depressed. As a coping mechanism, abuse of alcohol and/or drugs is possible, which can compound the problem further.

Scenario Five: Post-traumatic stress disorder

James, a 27-year-old city banker, was caught up in the July 2005 London bombings. He was on an underground tube train near King's Cross when the train carriage exploded next to where he was sitting. Luckily, James escaped with minor injuries, but he is still disturbed by the sights and sounds that he encountered immediately following the explosion. He has recurrent nightmares and says that he can hear the voices of the victims calling out as soon as he tries to go to sleep. James has been prescribed night sedation by his GP, but this does not appear to be working. Nowadays, he tends to stay indoors. James has not returned to work since this incident happened and he shudders at the idea of going underground to take a trip on a tube train.

PANIC DISORDER

'Panic disorder' is the term given for an attack of severe anxiety and fear that envelops the person at any time without any cause or stimulus (Smith 2000). The person could be carrying on with their daily activities when, suddenly, they can develop an overwhelming sense of panic for no apparent reason (Davies 2002). The person may feel as if they are losing control of their life and sometimes may feel as if they are experiencing a heart attack. They experience feelings such as palpitations, sweating, chest tightness and/or pain, trembling, dizziness, increased breathing, as if the autonomic nervous system has reacted spontaneously to a stressful situation but in the absence of any stressful situation. This could last for a matter of minutes but may be prolonged for much longer (Stuart 2002). At other times, the person may experience situational panic disorder, especially when they find themselves in a place or situation when attacks have happened previously. Panic disorder is more prevalent in females but can also be a part of the presentation in phobias or post-traumatic stress disorder.

Scenario Six: Panic disorder

Carole is a 17-year-old girl who will be sitting her A-level examinations in June. She is hoping to go on to university in September, where she will read psychology. Carole's parents are proud of her and have always made it clear to Carole that they expect her to do well. While studying one day, Carole was reflecting on her course work and the expectations her parents had of her. She suddenly found it hard to breathe and experienced a tight gripping-type pain in her chest. Her heart was pounding and she was trembling. This episode lasted for about ten minutes. Carole was taken to her local A & E, but no problems were detected. This recently happened again in the middle of the night. Carole woke up suddenly and experienced the same symptoms as before. Carole was taken to the A & E department but, again, no abnormalities were detected. While in A & E, Carole was seen and examined by a psychiatrist who diagnosed panic disorder. This was attributed to the current pressure that Carole was experiencing due to her studies and impending examinations.

THE TREATMENT OF ANXIETY DISORDERS

The treatment of anxiety disorders is variable and will be directly linked to the nature and severity of the anxiety being experienced by the person. As mentioned above, anxiety is one of the most treatable psychiatric disorders. However, it must also be remembered that anxiety may coexist in the presence of other psychological disorders, such as depression. All this information must be considered when treating anxiety disorders. It is suggested that a full assessment of needs is carried out prior to any treatment regimes being implemented in order to establish exactly what needs to be treated, why it needs to be treated and how it is going to be effectively dealt with (Donald *et al.* 2001). When considering the treatment of anxiety disorders, it is possible that some treatments can be used in conjunction with each other to attain and maintain maximum benefits.

RELAXATION TRAINING

'Relaxation training' (or 'relaxation technique', as it is also known) involves training the person about the importance of regular relaxation of the body's muscles and making the person more aware of their posture. This is beneficial in mild to moderate anxiety states because it allows respite to the already tense muscles and encourages the person to relax different areas of the body at different times (Stuart 2002). Initially, the person will need support and guidance to ensure the correct technique is being learned. Once this has been achieved, the person can continue this technique in their own time and can use this to their advantage.

BREATHING EXERCISES

When considering the anxiety cycle, breathing is one aspect that increases with exposure to a stressful stimulus. A problem associated with increased breathing is that of hyperventilation, where the body has a higher than needed level of oxygen. The person uses their abdominal muscles as opposed to the upper chest muscles. When the person encounters an anxious situation, it is essential that the breathing rate and rhythm are controlled. Compared to relaxation training, appropriate breathing exercises can be taught and can be used as necessary in dealing effectively with mild to moderate anxiety. The aim of breathing exercises is to make the person aware of the importance of their breathing pattern and to demonstrate the efficacy of this technique when faced with an anxious situation. However, it is essential that these are practised at least twice a day for up to 30 minutes at a time to gain optimum benefit (Trickett 1996). Once an acceptable technique has been learned and adopted, the person could practise these exercises, even while carrying out daily routines.

COUNSELLING

In dealing with mild anxiety and associated depression, the use of person-centred counselling is effective (Katona & Robertson 2000). This allows the person to explore the problems associated with the anxiety which he/she is currently experiencing. Central to the idea of person-centred counselling are the ideas of empathy, warmth, genuineness and unconditional positive regard, the latter being a method of allowing the person to openly discuss their thoughts and feelings without feeling intimidated or threatened (Thompson & Mathias 2000). However, it is essential that the person does not become dependent on the counsellor to provide all of the answers to their problems. If this happens, the counsellor should possess skills to intervene accordingly. Person-centred counselling usually occurs weekly, and the nature and severity of the anxiety state determines the duration of this intervention. This intervention can allow the person to explore their own thoughts and feelings surrounding their anxiety with a view to supporting problem-solving abilities (Parry 1996). As a result of this, the person should be able to adopt more capable ways of living, with or without the continued professional support of the mental health services.

SUPPORTIVE PSYCHOTHERAPY

This is the simplest form of psychotherapy and can be effective in treating mild to moderate anxiety (Shives & Isaacs 2002). It allows freedom of speech around the person concerning their problems and symptoms. Following disclosure by the person, it is the therapist who suggests coping methods related to dealing with problems. This is regarded as lessening the psychological load for the person with the intention of allowing them a reprieve from their worries. It also intends to boost the person's performance while emphasising the importance of adopting coping strategies. However, dependency on the therapist must always be discouraged as this would defeat the purpose of the therapy. Supportive psychotherapy engages the person, assists with the articulation of thoughts and feelings and encourages the development of their problem-solving abilities by means of reflection. It also encourages the person to be proactive as opposed to passive in dealing with problems; hence cooperation on the person's part is essential.

BEHAVIOUR THERAPY

It is suggested that behaviour therapy shows great benefits in dealing with phobias and obsessive-compulsive disorders. Behaviour therapy focuses on altering the reaction provoked by anxiety by means of acquiring new skills when dealing with perceived problems (Deakin 1993). This involves direct exposure to the problem, and it can be rapid (known as 'flooding') or gradual (known as 'desensitisation') (Davies & Armstrong 2002). The behaviour of the person is analysed, taking into account their thoughts and feelings before, during and after the incident. Positive reactions are reinforced with negative reactions being managed by further training and recognition of the stimulus that is causing the anxiety. The person is encouraged to take on some responsibility and ownership within behaviour therapy. This is done by keeping diaries and written evidence relating to activity schedules that the person has undertaken. From this, the person can develop a better understanding of the problems they are experiencing, and this assists both parties in effectively dealing with the presenting problems.

COGNITIVE BEHAVIOUR THERAPY

'Cognitive behavioural therapy' (or CBT) is a method of treatment that is often used in the treatment of severe anxiety disorder and post-traumatic stress disorder. CBT is defined as:

> any mode or therapy that attempts to change client's thinking, behaviours and affect through the use of pragmatic implementation of sound evidence (Rogers & Gournay 2002).

CBT relates to the patient's perception of the events that cause upset. The belief behind CBT is that it endeavours to improve the person's response to the anxiety-provoking situation by exploring the person's thoughts and feelings about the situation. It is used to explore problems in great depth to uncover any issues in order to deal with them appropriately. The aim of CBT is to reinforce acceptable reactionary behaviour and develop new coping skills towards the object causing anxiety. It also allows the person to review their circumstances in light of this new information in an attempt to improve their situation and dispel any fears.

PHARMACOLOGICAL INTERVENTIONS

Drug therapy can be used to combat feelings of anxiety in an attempt to improve the person's quality of life. It is worth remembering that the use of prescribed medication is not usually the first line of treatment, as other methods of care interventions will be considered initially. However, there are times when the use of prescribed drugs is indicated, especially when the level of anxiety is so great that it does not allow the person to act or think rationally, let alone function. Drugs can generally be employed at this time to help reduce the level of anxiety in order to facilitate relaxation in the person, or while allowing other interventions such as therapy to be carried out. Healy (2005) suggests the use of various categories of drugs that can be effective in combating anxiety states.

Benzodiazepine anxiolytic drugs such as diazepam (Valium) are commonly used, but media coverage in the late 1980s and early 1990s reported the addictive effects of such drugs. Benzodiazepines can be long-, short- or medium-acting drugs. However, they should be limited to the minimum dose for a specific duration and their efficacy subsequently reassessed.

Antidepressants can also be prescribed, namely selective serotonin reuptake inhibitors (SSRIs), tricyclic antidepressants (TCAs) and monoamine oxidase inhibitors (MAOIs). SSRIs are recognised for treating various anxiety disorders and are less addictive than benzodiazepines. TCAs were discovered in the 1950s and can be beneficial in treating panic disorder, since these drugs have a sedative component. MAOIs are effective in dealing with phobias, but these are seldom used. This is because they interact easily with other drugs and can also interact with certain foods containing yeast or meat extracts, for example Bovril, Marmite and Oxo, as well as mature cheese, pickled herring and plain chocolate. MAOIs are usually used as a last resort following the failure of all other drug therapy.

Beta-blockers are also used for the treatment of generalised anxiety disorder, but these drugs as a rule are used to treat high blood pressure and other associated cardiac problems. They are effective in blocking the lateral symptoms of anxiety such as trembling, increased heart rate etc. However, it must be pointed out that these drugs are ineffective when dealing with panic disorder (Healy 2005).

During drug interventions for any disorder, it is essential to remember that all drugs have side effects, some of which can be very unpleasant and frightening. They may lead to an exacerbation of an already recognised disorder, such as anxiety. It is imperative that a correct diagnosis is established before any drug therapy is initiated. While the person is receiving specific drug therapy, it is crucial that they are monitored and reviewed at regular intervals by a qualified health care professional to explore and determine the efficacy of the prescribed drug therapy. This, in turn, must be documented in the case notes (or other records relating to the person) by the health care professional.

CONCLUSION

Anxiety is inherent in everybody, and at times of crisis it can be beneficial to the person's welfare and, occasionally, survival. It can inform people as to what plan of action could be undertaken when in crisis, with positive or negative results. The effects of such results may teach the person new skills and knowledge, which they can use to their own benefit in the future.

However, problems may occur when a heightened level of anxiety is sustained over a period of time. This could be due to a physical exposure to a stressor, an imbalance of hormones within the body itself as a result of this prolonged exposure or other reasons. Subsequently, the body's nervous system continues to function, which could result in physical, psychological and emotional exhaustion. In the worst-case scenario, it could lead to death if not treated appropriately.

Treatments of anxiety disorders are many and varied and rely heavily on the signs and symptoms being reported and displayed by the person at that particular time. All treatments should be carefully considered, weighing up the advantages and disadvantages of the specific situation. Any changes relating to treatments must be specified and discussed with the individual in order to reassure the person, while identifying any further effects that may occur. Treatments must be recognised and repeatedly assessed for efficacy, taking into account the welfare of the person. If any drug therapy is prescribed, this must be prescribed by a relevant health care professional, who should view drug therapy as only part of a holistic approach to treating a person's physical, psychological and emotional problems.

REFERENCES

Ash J (1997) Behavioural psychotherapy. In Thomas B, Hardy S, Cutting P (eds), *Stuart and Sundeen's Mental Health Nursing: Principles and Practice*. Edinburgh, Mosby, pp. 453–470.

Barker P (1993) Stress and distress. In Wright H, Giddey M (eds), *Mental Health Nursing: From First Principles to Professional Practice*. Cheltenham, Stanley Thorne, pp. 103–115.

Davies M (2002) Interventions for anxiety, stress and depression: skills for primary care nurses. In Armstrong E (ed), *The Guide to Mental Health for Nurses in Primary Care*. Oxford, Radcliffe Medical Press, pp. 37–50.

Davies M, Armstrong E (2002) Anxiety, stress and related conditions. In Armstrong E (ed.), *The Guide to Mental Health for Nurses in Primary Care*. Oxford, Radcliffe Medical Press, pp. 27–36.

Deakin G (1993) Behavioural and cognitive-behavioural approaches. In Wright H, Giddey M (eds), *Mental Health Nursing. From First Principles to Professional Practice*. Cheltenham, Stanley Thorne, pp. 251–292.

Donald S, Lancaster R, Forster S (2001) The nurse as assessor. In Forster S (ed), *The Role of the Mental Health Nurse*. Cheltenham, Nelson Thornes, pp. 13–36.

Healy D (2005) *Psychiatric Drugs Explained* (4th edn.). London, Elsevier.

Katona C, Robertson M (2000) *Psychiatry at a Glance* (2nd edn.). Oxford, Blackwell Science.

Lovell K, Richards D (1997) Care of the survivor. In Thomas B, Hardy S, Cutting P (eds), *Stuart and Sundeen's Mental Health Nursing: Principles and Practice*. Edinburgh, Mosby, pp. 377–394.

Martin EA (ed) (2003) *Oxford Dictionary of Nursing* (4th edn.). Oxford, Oxford University Press.

Muir-Cochrane E (2003) The person who experiences anxiety. In Barker P (ed), *Psychiatric and Mental Health Nursing: The Craft of Caring*. London, Arnold Publishers, pp. 211–218.

Parry G (1996) Using research to challenge practice. In Heller T, Reynolds J, Gomm R, Muston R, Pattison S (eds), *Mental Health Matters: A Reader*. Basingstoke, Macmillan, pp. 282–289.

Puri BK (2000) Neurotic, stress-related and somatoform disorders. In Kumar P, Clark M (eds), *Saunders' Pocket Essentials of Psychiatry* (2nd edn.). Philadelphia, WB Saunders/Elsevier, pp. 115–128.

Rogers P, Gournay K (2002) Nurse therapy in forensic mental health. In Kettles A, Woods P, Collins P (eds), *Therapeutic Interventions for Forensic Mental Health Nurses*. London, Jessica Kingsley, pp. 151–164.

Semple D, Smyth R, Burns J, Darjee R, McIntosh A (2005) *Oxford Handbook of Psychiatry*. Oxford, Oxford University Press.

Seyle H (1956) *The Stress of Life*. New York, McGraw-Hill.

Shives LR, Isaacs A (2002) *Basic Concepts of Psychiatric–Mental Health Nursing* (5th edn.). Philadelphia, Lippincott Williams & Wilkins.

Smith LD (2000) Mental health problems. In Thompson T, Mathias P (eds), *Lyttle's Mental Health and Disorder* (3rd edn.). Edinburgh, Balliere Tindall, pp. 173–186.

Spielberger C (1987) Understanding stress and anxiety. In Martin P (ed) *Care of the Mentally Ill* (2nd edn.). Basingstoke, Macmillan Education.

Stuart G (ed) (2002) *Pocket Guide to Psychiatric Nursing* (5th edn.). St Louis, Mosby-Yearbook.

Thomas G (2004) *Anxiety Toolbox: Do You Put Your Life on Hold to Avoid the Situations that Scare You?* London, HarperCollins.

Thompson T, Mathias P (eds) (2000) *Lyttle's Mental Health and Disorder* (3rd edn.). Edinburgh, Balliere Tindall.

Trickett S (1996) *Coping with Anxiety and Depression*. London, Sheldon Press.

Van Wynsberghe D, Noback CR, Carola R (1995) *Human Anatomy and Physiology* (3rd edn.). New York, McGraw-Hill.

8 Mood Disorders Including Self-harm and Suicide

S. CLOUDSDALE

INTRODUCTION

This chapter will consider some of the descriptions and explanations of depression. It will look at some of the treatments available and will outline the theoretic standpoints that underpin certain explanations and treatment approaches.

All of us have differences in our moods. We can feel quite happy and at other times quite low in mood, or sad. This presents the majority of people with no significant problem. It is natural to feel happy or elated in response to precipitating events such as passing an examination or winning a prize or the birth of a baby; conversely, it is natural to feel low or sad when dealing with things such as a loss of job or the breakup of a relationship. The loss of a loved one to death provokes a special kind of sadness; this will be discussed later.

Some people, however, have to live with mood disturbances that are far beyond the norm in their length and profundity. There are two types of mood disorder that have been generally accepted; they are:

- unipolar depression
- bipolar depression.

UNIPOLAR DEPRESSION

In unipolar depression, the person feels only depressive symptoms. In bipolar depression, the person will experience a range of moods; this will stretch from feeling profoundly low in mood to feeling extremely elated (Stirling & Hellwell 1999). An important point to remember here is that these depths and range of moods do not necessarily correspond to a precipitating event in the person's life, although in some cases they can. Bereavement, feeling very sad after a person close to you has died, is a natural process that moves along at a pace unique to an individual. The

Caring for Adults with Mental Health Problems   Edited by I. Peate and S. Chelvanayagam
© 2006 John Wiley & Sons, Ltd

important thing is that, eventually, the process comes to an end and the individual accepts the loss and moves on with their lives. For some people, this process is protracted and they remain in a very low mood for a very long time.

People who have problems with mood disturbance or depression can show a collection of behaviours and ideas that form 'symptoms', that is they tend to be consistent from one person to another. They can be grouped as:

- emotional symptoms
- cognitive symptoms
- motivational symptoms
- somatic symptoms.

In the emotional or 'feelings' area, the person may indicate that they are feeling 'sad', 'low', 'helpless', 'unhappy', 'worried', 'useless' or 'guilty'. A person may find that these feelings alter in severity depending on the time of day with the most profound feelings happening in the morning with a lightening of mood later in the day. Along with these feelings can go a loss of satisfaction with occupations or pursuits that once gave them pleasure. Some people who enjoyed going out avoid doing so, and as a result become quite isolated. Eventually, this profound low mood will affect some biological functions, for example eating and enjoying sex; there will be a general loss or lowering of appetite (Rosenhan & Seligman 1995).

A person who is very low in mood will have recognisable cognitive (how they think – the process of thinking) symptoms. Such people tend to think of themselves in a very negative light and may have quite low self-esteem. They may think that they lack the qualities of a successful person and that they are inadequate. They may think that they are significantly less attractive, intelligent or generally talented or lacking in competence than other people. Figure 8.1 provides an example taken from a cognitive behavioural therapy session with a depressed client.

From the dialogue in Figure 8.1 it can be determined how low in esteem the patient is and how he finds it difficult to credit himself with success. The therapist is attempting to engage the client in an objective examination of the false assumptions that the client is burdened with in relation to his competence in hanging wallpaper. People who are in this low-mood nexus also believe that their future is one of hopelessness, and this view is very difficult to dislodge. People in this condition feel that their actions will have no positive outcome.

People have different levels of motivation; for example being quite enthusiastic about going on holiday and the need to prepare for this event. Going back to work on the Monday morning after our holiday will, for most people, not fill us with enthusiasm; however, the important thing is that we do go to work – we have enough motivation to get us there. People who are in a very low mood find it very difficult to get any task started. Some depressed people can be found just sitting motionless day after day. In the most severe cases, some people cannot

---

One person who papered their kitchen while very depressed gave the following account:

Therapist: Why didn't you rate wallpapering as a mastery experience?
Patient: Because the flowers didn't line up.
Therapist: You did, in fact, complete the job?
Patient: Yes.
Therapist: It's your kitchen?
Patient: No. I helped a neighbour do his kitchen.
Therapist: Did he do most of the work?
Patient: No. I really did almost all of it. He hadn't wallpapered before.
Therapist: Did anything else go wrong? Did you spill paste all over? Ruin a lot of wallpaper? Leave a big mess?
Patient: No, no. The only problem was that the flowers did not line up.
Therapist: So, since it was not perfect, you get no credit at all?
Patient: Well …yes.
Therapist: Just how far off was the alignment of the flowers?
Patient: (*holds out figures about 30 mm apart*) About that much.
Therapist: On each strip of paper?
Patient: No …on two or three pieces.
Therapist: Out of how many?
Patient: About 20 to 30.
Therapist: Did anyone else notice?
Patient: No. In fact, my neighbour thought it was great.
Therapist: Did your wife see it?
Patient: Yes. She admired the job.
Therapist: Could you see the defect when you stood back and looked at the whole wall?
Patient: Well …not really.
Therapist: So you have selectively attended to a real but small flaw in your effort to wallpaper. Is it logical that such a small defect should entirely cancel the credit you deserve?
Patient: Well, it was as good as it should have been.
Therapist: If your neighbour had done the same quality job in your kitchen, what would you say?
Patient: (*pause*) Pretty good job!

Figure 8.1 Narrative associated with cognitive behavioural therapy (adapted from Beck *et al.* 1979)

bring themselves to do things that are necessary to maintain life, such as eating and drinking. For the person who is depressed, every decision is a momentous one, even deciding whether to eat or to get dressed in the morning.

Somatic symptoms (symptoms of the body) are quite marked in severe depression. The most common one is loss of appetite leading to a significant reduction in weight. The person's sleep pattern is affected and they may complain of fitful sleep and waking up quite early in the morning. There is a marked loss of interest in sexual activity; men may experience erectile difficulties and women a lack of sexual arousal (Stirling & Hellwell 1999). As well as these symptoms, the depressed person can become susceptible to infections such as influenza.

BIPOLAR DEPRESSION

The other form of depression, known as bipolar (or manic) depression, will now be discussed. This is where the person has manic episodes as well as those of severe depression; so the person can go through a range of moods from severe depression to extreme elation.

The mood of a person in a manic state will be euphoric and elevated, however the most likely mood is one of irritability and the person may manifest this when their unrealistic plans are thwarted.

The thoughts that a person in this condition has are mood appropriate, that is they are exiting and grandiose. The person does not appreciate any limits to their ability and will seem oblivious to the consequences of their actions. One person who had inherited quite a lot of money spent the lot on hiring helicopters to fly her over the Scottish lochs. We may say that she was entitled to do what she wanted with her own money, but it did not stop there, and the person went into severe debt. The person in this state may have ideas running through their mind faster than they can write them down or even express them verbally. They may have strange ideas that they have a special purpose or mission or may even be a messenger of God.

Manic behaviour is hyperactive; this means that the person will engage in activities at a breakneck speed. This behaviour can be ill judged, such as unsafe casual sexual activity or behaviour that can put their employment in jeopardy, such as not turning up for work or neglecting their tasks. The activities of a person in this condition can be intrusive and demanding and the ordinary, everyday etiquette of social interaction will seem to be forgotten by the person. Their behaviour can be quite coarse, such as using profanities or exposing themselves. Spending any time with people in this condition can be quite tiring.

Physically, this will all be quite exhausting for the person thus affected, after a few days, their physical exhaustion will slow them down. They may become less active, dehydrated and undernourished. Treatment will be addressed after the cause of depression has been discussed.

CAUSES OF DEPRESSION

An analysis of the causes of depression could fill an entire book; therefore, a brief outline of the major theories will be provided. These theories are generally divided into biological and psychological factors.

At first sight, the person who is grieving and a depressive person look rather similar; both seem to be drained and withdrawn. This similarity prompted thinkers such as Sigmund Freud to suggest that both states may have the same cause. As mourning is motivated by loss, could depression by motivated by some other form of loss? Freud (1917) noticed that not all his depressed clients had experienced an actual loss but behaved as if they had. Freud's hypothesis was that the cause of depression is bound up with early childhood experiences; in his /her childhood, depressed person will have developed an intense love for another person that is undermined and leads to disappointment in that person. The libidinal energy is released, but, unlike mourning where there is a gradual detachment from the lost person and an eventual opening up to others as the grieving process subsides, the depressed child identifies with the lost person and incorporates the lost person within themselves. The rage and anger that is normally expressed outwardly towards the lost person is now directed inwardly toward the person's own sense of self. It is felt that it is this that creates the low self-esteem of the depressed person. A child that has been deprived of love or has been abused will have had their love undermined and in a sense will have 'lost' the significant love object. This sense of self worth will have been greatly damaged, whereas in 'normal' grieving the sense of self worth is usually intact and survives the loss (Stirling & Hellwell 1999).

The biological theory for depression centres on the chemical make-up of the human body, and of the brain in particular. Modern theories concentrate on the neurotransmitting chemicals in the brain and particularly on the alteration in the number and sensitivity of receptors. Three monoamine neurotransmitter systems have been identified; these are noradrenaline, serotonin (or 5-HT) and dopamine. Analysis of the brain tissue of those depressed who have killed themselves has indicated a lower than normal level of 5-HT. This, along with the discovery of increased receptor sites, indicates that a low level of 5-HT activity is most likely the cause of depression in the majority of people who suffer from it. Medication, such as fluoxetine hydrochloride (Prozac), acts to block the receptor sites of 5-HT and, therefore, raise the level of serotonin and, as a consequence, lift the client's mood.

Research that has been carried out on identical and non-identical twins gives weight to the genetic and, therefore, biological explanation for depression. The treatment of bipolar depression involves the use of lithium carbonate, a naturally occurring chemical that is deficient in such clients; this also gives credence to the biological explanation for depression.

A more recent explanation for the occurrence of depression has been called SAD (seasonal affective disorder). Some people report that their depressive symptoms are much worse in the winter months and not so pronounced, or entirely absent, during the spring and summer months. The amount of light available is the variable here. A study by Rosenthal et al. (1984) showed that depressive symptoms in these people were associated with sunlight and temperature: when some of the people in his study moved to the south of the United States of America from the north, their symptoms lessened. When they travelled north in the winter months, their symptoms worsened. Indeed, the use of light therapy where strong lighting is used to artificially lengthen the days in winter has been found to produce significant improvement in the mood of these people (Rosenthal et al. 1984).

The accepted statistics for prevalence of depression (i.e. what proportion of the population is suffering from depression at any one time) is 8.56%. The figures are 10.05% for women and 6.1% for men (Royal College of Psychiatrists 2001). It is interesting that the figures for women are higher than those for men; you will find that this phenomenon is repeated amongst most reports you may look at. There are various explanations for this, but the most convincing is that more women than men report depressive symptoms to their doctors. There may be several reasons for this. It is thought that men are far more reluctant to go to their GP with depressive symptoms and see such attendance as some form of weakness on their part (Norman & Ryrie 2004). The study by Norman and Ryrie found that there was a difference in the prevalence of depression between urban UK and Ireland (12.8% and 17.1% respectively) and urban Spain (2.6%). Sociologists put forward the view that such differences are due to cultural reasons (Giddens 1992).

GENERAL SUPPORT

The key aim is to try and build a therapeutic relationship with the person, that is a relationship that supports and helps the person as they go through this depressive process. This can be done by engaging with the person and listening to what they have to say. This engagement may be difficult if they are withdrawn and not speaking. However, the person will recognise a positive approach towards them and will appreciate it. This is evidenced by the comments of some clients later on; many have said that they felt supported by the helping person's presence even if not very much was said. It is important to be non-judgemental towards people who are depressed. It may be a temptation to think, 'Why don't you just snap out of it?' or 'I've been through personal tragedy; why can't you pull yourself together as I did?' Such thoughts are natural; however, if you reflect on how you dealt with your own feelings of sadness or sad events, you will remember that it was not quite that straightforward and will recall those people who were near to you and the level of support that they gave you. The person who is depressed will need a great deal of support and kindness (Norman & Ryrie 2004).

TREATMENT

Some people who are depressed will need some form of medical or psychological treatment to help them overcome their present condition. The form of treatment will follow on from the particular theory of causation of the condition. Most people with reactive depressions (i.e. in relation to a precipitating event) may receive a course in counselling or some other form of talking therapy (see Chapter 14 in this book). In this discursive process, the person will have an opportunity to examine the events that are making them feel so sad and to put them into perspective. The transcript in Table 8.1 is an example of one such approach, cognitive behavioural therapy (CBT); other approaches may be a more general discursive process based on a psychodynamic explanation of depression (see below).

People who are more profoundly depressed may, especially if there is no known precipitating event, have some form of medical intervention, such as antidepressant medication or in the most severe cases a form of physical therapy known as

Table 8.1 Some antidepressant medication (Adapted from Rethink 2006)

Pharmacological name	Brand name
amitriptyline hydrochloride	Triptizol Lentizol
clomipramine	Anafranil
dothiepin hydrochloride	Prothiaden
doxepin	Sinequan
imipramine	Tofranil
citalopram	Cipramil
fluoxetine	Prozac
paroxetine	Seroxat
sertraline	Lustral

electroconvulsive therapy (ECT). This form of therapy, where electricity is passed over part of the brain, helps to lift the mood of the person with depression quite markedly; however, it is a form of therapy that is opposed by some users of the mental health service and some mental health practitioners because of its side effect on short-term memory loss and the controversy associated with its use.

Most people will receive treatment for depression in the form of antidepressant medication. These are given to improve the mood of the depressed person. Their action is upon the neurotransmitters within the brain; too little of these transmitters may cause depression (Norman & Ryrie 2004). The action of these drugs helps block the reuptake of these transmitters and, therefore, leaves more of them available. The result may be a lifting of the person's mood. Table 8.1 above details some of the more familiar antidepressant drugs.

All of the above drugs are used to combat low mood and depression. They may need up to two weeks of administration before they start working. They need to be taken in the right dosage for between six months and several years (Rethink 2006).

SELF-HARM AND SUICIDE

Some people seek to harm themselves when they are severely depressed or, in some cases, kill themselves. It can be quite difficult to understand why people seek to do these things to themselves; therefore, it may be better to have a person who has these thoughts and tendencies to speak for themselves.

Scenario: Rosalyn (18 years old)

I thought that my self-injuring was just something I could do occasionally, without any major consequences. Unfortunately, I was dreadfully wrong. As the months went by, I became addicted to the sensation that my self-injury gave me. I began to collect scars on my arms and legs, ankles, thighs, hips and anywhere I could find.

I secretly enjoyed the scars and would sometimes spend hours just looking at them from different angles. It is so contradictory because I was ashamed to let anyone else see them.

The day I knew I had to get help was about a year and a half into my self-injury. I knew I was severely depressed and couldn't help myself, no matter how much I wanted to. I am in a group at the personality disorder clinic that teaches me how to try and regulate powerful emotions.

I have been seeing a psychologist for the past year. He cares deeply about me and goes up and beyond his call of duty to make sure I stay safe.

I want to believe that I will get through this trial in my life. I want to believe that I will recover from self-injuring. I still struggle every day of my life but in the end it will be worth it (adapted from Lifesigns 2006).

The above is an example of how someone who is severely depressed may seek to harm themselves. What must be remembered here is that the self-harming behaviour helps the person deal with their depression, negative self-image and stress. Therefore, the self-harming behaviour is symptomatic of an underlying unhappiness.

It is difficult to understand why people go further and kill themselves. There is a societal prohibition on self-killing that stretches far back in time; however, suicide was not condemned in the West until the fourth century CE, when St. Augustine proclaimed it a crime because it violated the sixth commandment 'Though shalt not kill'. It was not until 1961 that suicide (and attempted suicide) ceased to be a criminal offence in the UK.

In 2003, there were recorded 18.1 deaths per 100,000 of the population from suicide; men are four times as likely than women to kill themselves, but three times as many women as men make suicide attempts that do not result in death (Mind 2006). This may seem to be a relatively low number; however, each death may have been preventable and each one is the centre of a family tragedy. Depressed people are the single group that is most at risk of suicide; however, the majority of people who are depressed do not go on to kill themselves. Approximately, 80% of suicidal people are severely depressed. Those depressed people who ultimately kill themselves do so at a rate that is 25 times higher than the general population (Rosenhan & Seligman 1995).

There may be several explanations for this phenomenon. Self-killing is such a complicated behaviour that no one model or concept can encompass it; therefore, we will have to look at some of the main models of suicide.

NEUROBIOLOGICAL MODELS

Studies show that risk of suicide is greater for identical twins than it is for non-identical twins (Baldessarini & Hennen 2004). It has been found that there are low levels of serotonin in people who have killed themselves (Coryell & Schlesser 2001). This suggests that there are biochemical explanations for the very low mood of those who kill themselves and that there is a certain heritable risk of being predisposed to self-killing; the fact that identical twins are at greater risk (as twins) than non-identical twins demonstrates this.

SOCIOCULTURAL MODELS

These models state that society can have a direct or indirect influence on those who are depressed or suicidal. Media coverage of famous suicides can spark an increase in suicide attempts, far more than coverage of non-celebrities (Gould 2001). Media reports of natural deaths of famous people do not spark an increase in suicide attempts. These finding suggest that there are societal influences at work.

Émile Durkheim (1858–1917) was a seminal thinker in relation to the analysis of suicide. He looked at such questions as 'Why do people kill themselves?' and 'What sort of people kill themselves?' and 'In what circumstances do they do this?' He developed a theory of three distinct categories of suicide:

- Egoistic: This is where people with no or little ties to family, society or the community generally kill themselves.
- Altruistic: This is where people kill themselves, or put themselves in the way of great danger, for the good of others. Examples of this are those who sacrifice themselves to save their children, or other people, from burning buildings, honour self-killing such as ritualised self-killing amongst Japanese people and others who follow their example.
- Anomic: This is where suicide is triggered by some form of sudden change in a person's personal circumstances and their relation to society. An example of this is the higher-than-normal suicide rate in post-Second World War Germany and in Russia after the fall of communism. A more up-to-date example is that of the higher rates of suicide in rural China. China has one of the fastest-growing economies in the world, and this has resulted in mass migration to the cities from rural areas. In these rural areas, suicide has become one of the main causes of death (Phillips *et al.* 2002).

When considering these issues, we must remember that these theories do not account for how individuals react to changing events; the majority of people who go through major life-changing events do not kill themselves.

PSYCHOLOGICAL MODELS

Suicide has been viewed as a retaliation for some hurt done as well as to instil feelings of guilt in others. Related to this is the theory that it is designed to force love from others on the part of a dependent partner (Rosenhan & Seligman 1995). It is, however, predominantly viewed as a bid to avoid unacceptable feelings. These are the sort of feelings that may be expressed by the clients requiring care; these feelings are the types of feelings that have been dealt with above. An example of this is the suicide note to her husband that was left by the novelist Virginia Woolf, who killed herself by drowning on the 28th March 1941. In the letter, she alludes to a functional mental illness when she talks about 'hearing voices'. The suicide rate amongst those who 'hear voices' is significantly higher than the general population (Mind 2006). These people are trying to avoid or escape from the symptoms of an illness that has become unacceptable to them (Figure 8.2).

Dearest

I feel certain I am going mad again. I feel we can't go through another of these terrible times. And I shan't recover this time. I begin to hear voices, and I can't concentrate. So I am doing what seems the best thing to do. You have given me the greatest possible happiness. You have been in every way all that anyone could be. I don't think two people could have been happier till this terrible disease came. I can't fight it any longer. I know that I am spoiling your life, that without me you could work, and you will I know. You see I can't even write this properly. I can't read. What I want to say is I owe all the happiness in my life to you. You have been entirely patient with me and incredibly good. I want to say that everybody knows it. If anybody could have saved me it would have been you. Everything has gone from me but the certainty of your goodness. I can't go on spoiling your life any longer. I don't think two people could have been happier than we have been.

V.

Figure 8.2 Virginia Woolf's suicide note (Quoted from pp 400–401, Briggs J (2005) Virginia Woolf: An Inner life. Orlando Fl, Harcourt)

Baumeister (1990) holds that people are at a significantly greater risk of suicide when they set themselves goals that are unrealistic and unattainable. When they fail to achieve these goals, they may indulge in self-blaming and view themselves as being unworthy. Suicide rates are higher in societies that have high expectations of achievement (Abela *et al.* 2006). The perfectionist, that is a person who sets extremely high standards for themselves, has a higher risk of suicide than those who do not have such high expectations.

Hopelessness is a strong predictor of suicidal behaviour. Hopelessness is the expectation that life will be no better in the future than it is now, and that it will never develop into something more fulfilling, and it is rather awful now from the perspective of the suicidal person. These high levels of hopelessness indicate a risk of suicide that is four times higher than that of the general population (Brown *et al.* 2000).

The question that all this raises is: 'How can suicide be prevented?' There is a common myth that talking about suicidal intentions will make the matter worse. This could not be further from the truth: giving people a place and time to talk about their self-harming or suicidal ideas will give them an opportunity to break out of a cycle of secrecy and isolation; it also gives the helping agent a better chance to assess the level of risk that the person is presenting (Norman & Ryrie 2004). Most people are ambivalent in their suicidal ideation, that is thinking about self-killing, and allowing them to talk about their feelings will help them explore this. Some other myths are highlighted in Table 8.2 below.

It must be remembered that most (but not all) people who are contemplating suicide are suffering from a mental illness. If the person's depression is reduced or lessened, the suicide risk will diminish.

An accepted strategy for preventing suicide is a threefold model implemented by Shneidman (1987):

1. Reduce the intense psychological pain.
2. Help the person see options other than continued suffering.
3. Encourage the person to pull back, even a little, from the self-destructive act.

A scenario taken from Shneidman illustrates this technique in action (Figure 8.3).

The example is similar in approach to the example shown in Figure 8.1 and draws on a cognitive method for helping such people examine, in an objective way, their ideas and feelings about suicide.

Currently, there is a focus on the reduction of suicide. The present Government has set a target that has developed into a climate of 'risk assessment and management' within clinical settings (Department of Health 1999). This has culminated in the doctrine of 'close observation' as the preferred method within such clinical settings. Close observation or 'continuous observation' means that the person is

Table 8.2 Some common myths and contrary evidence associated with suicide (adapted from Fremouw et al. 1990)

Common myth	Contrary evidence
People who discuss suicide will not actually commit suicide.	Up to three quarters of those who take their own lives communicate their intention beforehand.
Suicide is committed without warning.	People usually give many warnings, such as saying that the world would be better off without them or making unexpected and inexplicable gifts of highly valued possessions.
Suicidal people want to die.	Most people who commit suicide appear to be ambivalent about their own deaths. Most people are grateful after suicide is prevented.
People who attempt suicide by low-lethal means (i.e. methods that are insufficient to kill them) are not serious about killing themselves.	Many people are not well informed about pill dosages or human anatomy. Because of this, people who really want to die sometimes make non-lethal attempts.

A wealthy college student was single, pregnant and suicidal, with a clearly formed plan. The only solution she could think of besides suicide was never to have become pregnant, even to be virginal again.

I took out a sheet of paper and began to widen her blinkers (sic). I said something like, 'Now, let's see: You could have an abortion here locally.' She responded, 'I couldn't do that.' I continued, 'You could go away and have an abortion.' 'I couldn't do that.' 'You could bring the baby to term and keep the baby.' 'I couldn't do that.' 'You could have the baby adopted.' Further options were similarly dismissed. When I said, 'You can always commit suicide, but there is no need to do that today', there was no response. 'Now,' I said. 'Let's look at this list and rank them in order of your preference, keeping in mind that none of them is optimal.'

Just drawing up the list had a calming effect. The student's drive to kill herself receded, and she was able to rank the list even though she found something wrong with each item. But an important goal had been achieved: she had been pulled back from the brink.

Figure 8.3 Preventing suicide (adapted from Shneidman 1987)

observed at all times until an assessment is made that determines whether the risk of suicide has been reduced. The benefit of such close observation is that it provides an opportunity for the carer to develop a therapeutic relationship with the client; however, the experience reported by clients is that such observation is restricting, punishing, humiliating and far from therapeutic (Fletcher 1999). Methods have to be developed that allow an individual who is suicidal to be cared for without compromising their autonomy. Close observation is still to be used in emergencies where the risk of self-killing is imminent. An alternative to this is what Cutcliffe and Barker (2002) call 'engagement and inspiring hope'. They define 'close observation' as limiting the role of the carer to that of a custodian with little therapeutic value. They describe this process as one of forming a relationship, conveying acceptance and tolerance, listening and understanding. They point out that if a sense of being valued is conveyed by the carer the client will respond by opening up to the carer and a therapeutic relationship can begin. This process of 'engagement' can inspire hope and expectation in the client, something that they may have been lacking during their illness. In a study of what relatives found hope-inspiring, Talseth *et al.* (2001) outlined six themes:

1. being seen as a human being
2. participating in an I–you relationship
3. trusting staff, treatment and care
4. feeling trusted by staff
5. being consoled
6. entering into hope.

These can apply equally to the client or their relative. It will be important for the carer to listen and to accept that the person who is feeling this way may be angry and frustrated; the carer's task is to help the client explore their feelings and to gain a more positive outlook on their future.

CONCLUSION

This chapter has looked at the definition of various types of depression, its causes and some of the treatments available to people living with the condition. Those who are depressed, especially at the level of self-harming or suicide, want to be treated with respect, acceptance and tolerance. Carers must strive to understand what the cause of the person's depression might be and why they may be using self-harming behaviour or entertain thoughts of suicide as a coping mechanism. Lastly, those who work with people who are depressed, especially if that depressed person is self-harming or suicidal, must have some form of support to help them manage their own anxiety, frustration and anger. Being in a therapeutic relationship with a client is challenging and can also be frustrating and anger-producing; however, the privilege of journeying with a client along this dark and labyrinthine pathway to a brighter place can be immensely rewarding.

REFERENCES

Abela JRZ, Webb CA, Wagner C, Ho M-HR, Adams P (2006) The role of self-criticism, dependency, and hassles in the course of depressive illness: a multiwave longitudinal study, http://psp.sagepub.com/cgi/content/abstract/32/3/328, accessed 12 July 2006.

Baldessarini RJ, Hennen J (2004) Genetics of suicide: an overview. *Harvard Review of Psychiatry* **12**(1): 1–13.

Baumeister RF (1990) Suicide as escape from self. *Psychological Review* **97**(1): 90–113.

Beck AT, Rush AJ, Shaw BF, Emery G (1979) *Cognitive Therapy of Depression*. New York, Guilford Press.

Briggs J (2005) *Virginia Woolf: An Inner Life*. Orlando, FL, Harcourt.

Brown GK, Beck AT, Steer RA, Grisham JR (2000) Risk factors for suicide in psychiatric outpatients: a 20-year prospective study. *Journal of Consulting and Clinical Psychology* **68**(3): 371–377.

Coryell PT, Schlesser M (2001) The dexamethasone suppression test and suicide prevention. *American Journal of Psychiatry* **158**(5): 748–753.

Cutcliffe JR, Barker P (2002) Considering the care of the suicidal client and the case for 'engagement and inspiring hope' or 'observations'. *Journal of Psychiatric and Mental Health Nursing* **9**(5): 611–621.

Department of Health (1999) *National Service Framework for Mental Health: Modern Standards and Service Models*. London, The Stationery Office.

Fletcher RF (1999) The process of constant observation: perspectives of staff and suicidal patients. *Journal of Psychiatric and Mental Health Nursing* **6**(1): 9–14.

Fremouw W, DePerczel M, Ellis TE (1990) *Suicide Risk: Assessment and Response*. New York, Pergamon Press.

Freud S (1917) Mourning and meloncholia. In Strachey S (ed), *The Standard Edition of the Complete Psychological Works of Sigmund Freud*. London, Hogarth Press, 1962, volume 14, pp. 243–258.

Giddens A (1992) *Sociology*. Oxford, Polity Press.

Gould MS (2001) Suicide and the media. *Annals of the New York Academy of Sciences* **932**(April): 200–221.

LifeSIGNS (2006) LifeSIGNS self injury awareness booklet, http://www.google.com/u/ LifeSIGNS?q=Rosalyn&sa=Search&domains=selfharm.org&sitesearch=selfharm.org, accessed 19 July 2006.

Mind (2006) Mind features, http://www.mind.org.uk/information/factsheet/suicide/, accessed 18 July 2006.

Norman I, Ryrie I (2004) *The Art and Science of Mental Health Nursing*. Maidenhead, Open University Press.

Phillips MR, Li X, Zhanh Y (2002) Suicide rates in China: 1995–99. *Lancet* **359**(9309): 835–840.

Rethink (2006) Antidepressants, http://www.rethink.org/living_with_mental_illness/ treatment_and_therapy/medication/antidepressants/index.html, accessed 12 July 2006.

Rosenhan L, Seligman MEP (1995) *Abnormal Psychology*. London, WW Norton.

Rosenthal NE, Sack DA, Gillin JC, Lewy AJ, Goodwin EK, Davenport Y, *et al.* (1984) Seasonal affective disorder: a description of the syndrome and preliminary findings with light therapy. *Archives of General Psychiatry* **41**(1): 72–80.

Royal College of Psychiatrists (2001) Depression, http://www.rcpsych.ac.uk/pdf/ Depression.pdf, accessed 12 July 2006.

Shneidman ES (1987) A psychological approach to suicide. In VandenBos GR, Bryant BK (eds), *Cataclysms, Crises and Catastrophes: Psychology in Action*. Washington, American Psychological Association.

Stirling D, Hellwell SE (1999) *Psychopathology*. London, Routledge.

Talseth A, Gilji F, Norberg A (2001) Being met – a passageway to hope for relatives of patients at risk of committing suicide: a phenomenological hermeneutic study. *Archives of Psychiatric Nursing* **15**(6): 249–256.

9 Eating Disorders

S. CHELVANAYAGAM

INTRODUCTION

This chapter aims to provide an understanding and knowledge of eating disorders. It will describe the different types of eating disorders, and their causes, features, care and treatment approaches.

The media, and in particular television, has repeatedly focused on weight and shape. Recently, there has been much television coverage involving both the general public and celebrities describing their weight problems and taking part in a variety of diet and exercise regimes. These television programmes and images all reinforce the widely held belief that 'thin is beautiful', so much so that even girls as young as eight years old have reported feeling they are overweight (Robinson 2000).

Eating disorders are perceived to only affect females; however, estimated figures show that 10–33% of people with an eating disorder are male (Paterson 2004). The important point to stress when discussing 'eating disorders' is that this term does not reflect the complex psychological issues that precipitate and perpetuate these disorders.

Generally, eating disorders occur predominantly in Western societies (countries that are industrialised) (Bhugra *et al.* 2000) where there is more emphasis on the desire to be slim and that being slim denotes being beautiful. In some African and Asian countries, the opposite is true, in that weight symbolises beauty, and therefore the more overweight a person is, the more beautiful they are perceived to be (Furnham & Adam-Saib 2001). However, when people from these countries travel to Western societies and have children, it has been noted that these children can develop eating disorders (Furnham & Adam-Saib 2001; Bhugra *et al.* 2000).

DEFINING EATING DISORDERS

A person who has an eating disorder has a disturbance of eating habits or weight control behaviour with strong beliefs of what being overweight represents. This disturbance results in significant impairment of physical health or psychosocial

Caring for Adults with Mental Health Problems   Edited by I. Peate and S. Chelvanayagam
© 2006 John Wiley & Sons, Ltd

functioning but should not be due to a general physical disorder or other mental illness (Fairburn & Harrison 2003). The three main eating disorders are:

- anorexia nervosa
- bulimia nervosa
- binge eating disorder.

Each condition will be separately discussed due to the differing nature of the conditions and their treatment and management.

ANOREXIA NERVOSA

The first medical reports of anorexia nervosa were by Dr Richard Morton (an English physician) in 1689. He referred to the disorder as 'nervous consumption', but it was not until 1868 that Sir William Gull (an English physician) and Dr Charles Lasègue (a French physician) provided the term 'anorexia nervosa'. Their descriptions of the disorder are still used today. However, it was not until after 1960, when Dr Hilda Bruch (a German-born American psychiatrist) provided further details regarding the psychological aspects of anorexia nervosa combined with the physical features recorded by Gull and Lasègue, that anorexia nervosa was recognised as a distinct disorder (Fairburn & Brownell 2002). A literal translation of the term means a 'loss of appetite due to nervous reasons', which is misleading as the person does not lose their appetite but strictly restricts their food intake (Eating Disorders Association 2006a).

Anorexia nervosa is generally diagnosed in females, with men accounting for 10% of cases. However, community-based studies of both anorexia nervosa and bulimia nervosa suggest that there is one male case to every six female cases (Braun *et al.* 1999). As it is deemed a condition that affects teenage girls, health care professionals may not recognise anorexia nervosa in men (Duker & Slade 2003; Peate 2001). Men are often afraid to speak about their weight problems and may present to a health care professional with complications from the disorder, such as joint pain due to excessive exercising. In addition, most health care services are geared towards females (Paterson 2004; Peate 2001). Anorexia nervosa usually occurs during adolescence and affects 0.7% of teenage girls (Fairburn & Harrison 2003).

It has frequently been stated that the person with anorexia nervosa tends to come from the professional (social class 1, e.g. doctors, dentists and lawyers) and intermediate (social class 2, e.g. nurses and teachers) classes (O'Donnell 2002). Although this has been disputed, McClelland and Crisp (2001) found that when they examined the class status of women presenting with anorexia nervosa at their specialist clinic over the past 33 years:

- 67.5% came from social classes 1 and 2
- 21% came from social class 3 (skilled, e.g. clerical workers)
- 10.8% came from social classes 4 (semi-skilled, e.g. postal workers, telephone operators) and 5 (unskilled, e.g. cleaners, labourers).

There also appears to be a strong genetic link. Studies of twins have shown that for those who develop anorexia nervosa, 65% of identical twins both have anorexia nervosa, compared to 32% of non-identical twins. In respect of other female siblings of the person with anorexia nervosa, 6–10% have also been diagnosed (Semple *et al.* 2005).

Features of anorexia nervosa

A person will be diagnosed with anorexia nervosa if they have the following features (Norman & Ryrie 2004):

- low bodyweight, i.e. a body mass index (BMI) score of 17.5 (kgm^2) or less, or 15% or more lower than expected for age and height
- self-induced weight loss – vomiting, purging, excessive exercise, use of appetite suppressants and avoidance of 'fattening' foods
- body-image distortion – fear of fatness, overvalued ideas, imposed low-weight threshold
- amenorrhoea: absence of menstrual cycle; men will report a gradual loss of libido due to lowering of their testosterone.

Low body weight

The person with anorexia nervosa will present as very thin; they can be as low in weight as 30 kg (approximately 5 st). However, their weight is usually concealed by layers of clothes or baggy oversized clothes. They may also wear several layers of clothes as they feel cold constantly and can suffer from hypothermia (abnormally low body temperature). The skin will appear dry and they may have hair loss but their body may be covered with a layer of fine downy hair known as lanugo hair (Murphy & Manning 2003).

The BMI is a measurement that calculates whether a person is the correct weight for their height, and this will be recorded when a person is seen by a nurse or doctor. The BMI is calculated by dividing the patient's weight (in kilograms – kg) by their height in metres squared (m^2). A normal BMI score is 20–25 (kgm^2); someone who is underweight would have a score of 17.5–20 (kgm^2) and a person with anorexia nervosa would have a BMI score of below 17.5 (kgm^2) (Murphy & Manning 2003).

Self-induced weight loss

Anorexia nervosa usually begins after starting a diet, possibly with a group of friends (Hetherington 2000). However, whereas the friends stop dieting, the person with anorexia nervosa continues to diet, eating fewer and fewer calories and using a range of techniques to lose weight. Therefore, they avoid fattening foods such as sweets, biscuits, cakes and crisps, which contain predominantly carbohydrates and fats. Gradually, they reduce the intake of all foods, even fluids. So they may only eat half a carrot a day and drink water. After eating, they may make themselves vomit to avoid gaining weight or may use purgatives (laxatives or diuretics) to eliminate the foods and fluids from their body. The person with anorexia nervosa will also exercise excessively, especially after eating. This may mean several visits to the gym each day or jogging everywhere they go (Barker 2003). Appetite suppressants may be obtained from private diet clinics or they may take amphetamines to suppress their appetite and to give them greater energy to exercise more frequently. Therefore, it can be observed that some individuals will take drastic actions to lose weight. They will decide how much weight they aim to lose each day and set strict targets, which they will endeavour to attain. So they may weigh themselves several times a day (Kneisl *et al.* 2004).

Body-image distortion

It is widely believed that the person with anorexia nervosa does not see that they are thin but reports that they see themselves as overweight. However, people who have experienced anorexia nervosa state that this is not the case. They state that they are fully aware they are underweight but can also still feel huge and so have these two contradictory thoughts simultaneously (Chisholm 2002). They may also view their weight loss as an accomplishment (as it shows that they have control over their bodies) and not an affliction; therefore, there is limited motivation to change (Clark-Stone 2003).

People with anorexia nervosa are said to have overvalued ideas regarding weight and shape. This means that they feel that people are judged by how they look and being thin is good, whereas being overweight is bad (Murphy & Manning 2003). Their self-esteem is strongly linked to their weight; they feel happier when they lose weight but desolate when they gain or do not lose weight (Eby & Brown 2005).

Amenorrhoea

In females, one of the first questions a nurse or doctor may ask is whether the person's periods have stopped; usually this is the case. Sometimes, the periods stop before significant weight loss occurs. This can then motivate the person with anorexia nervosa to continue with the weight loss (there is a belief that one of the reasons this disorder occurs is that the female is trying to avoid growing into a woman). The commencement of the menstrual cycle means the process has began. If the female can halt this process by weight loss, this provides her with the motivation to continue in the hope that her maturity into womanhood can be stopped (Barker 2003).

Causes of anorexia nervosa

It is important to remember that, although many people who develop anorexia nervosa and bulimia do so following dieting, dieting itself does not cause an eating disorder. Hetherington (2000) asserts that it may be the trigger but that there is usually a range of other factors which precipitate the occurrence of the disorder.

The person who develops anorexia nervosa is often described as a perfectionist who is very self-critical. They may also be described as high achievers, working hard at school to achieve good grades. They have a strong desire to please others and therefore have often been obedient children. The person usually has low self-esteem with symptoms of depression or anxiety. They may be socially withdrawn, have a distorted body image (due to previous dietary issues or comments from family members) with a lack of sense of identity and wanting to regress back into childhood. The restriction of food may be motivated by severe self-discipline, competitiveness and a wish to punish themselves (Eating Disorders Association 2006a).

Ballet and fashion modelling are said to be some of the professions that can predispose a person to anorexia nervosa due to the need to be physically fit and very slim. However, it is not known whether a person who may be at risk of developing anorexia nervosa is attracted to these professions or whether the demands of these professions in some way provokes a desire to be overly thin and so precipitates the development of anorexia nervosa (Fairburn & Brownell 2002). The family of the person with anorexia nervosa has been described as overprotective, very rigid, with a lack of conflict resolution, preoccupation with food, obsessive and perfectionist traits and high expectations of all members of the family (Gelder *et al.* 2001). There may also be a history of childhood physical or sexual abuse, particularly seen in males (Paterson 2004).

Care and treatment

As mentioned above, the person with anorexia nervosa is frequently reluctant to seek help as they feel that they now have control over their body. Usually it is the parent who brings their child to the doctor. The person with anorexia needs to recognise that they need help and have motivation to change their behaviour. This can be a very frightening period for them; so they need support and empathy to enable them to accept help and treatment.

The National Institute for Health and Clinical Excellence (NICE) is an organisation that provides guidelines on treatment and management for a range of physical and mental health conditions (NICE 2004). These guidelines have been formulated by examining relevant research and talking to expert clinicians to ensure that a range of effective interventions are recommended. The NICE guidelines for eating disorders regarding appropriate care and treatment have been incorporated into this chapter.

Most people with anorexia nervosa will receive out-patient treatment as long as their weight is not dangerously low. The treatment will be in the form of psychological treatments such as cognitive behavioural therapy (CBT), interpersonal psychotherapy or family therapies (see Chapter 14 of this book). Interpersonal psychotherapy focuses on the problems the person experiences and the effect on their current functioning (Kirby *et al.* 2004). Cognitive behavioural therapy will address and challenge some of their beliefs about food and weight. Family therapy will help to address some of the underlying familial issues or conflicts that may have contributed to the person's development of anorexia nervosa.

These psychological treatments should be of at least six months' duration. Dietary counselling by a dietician will also occur and will help the person eat appropriate foods to gain weight and also provide education about nutrition. NICE (2004) does not recommend the use of drug treatments unless there is a clear indication of a separate mental health condition that requires treatment, for example if the person has a depressive illness as well as anorexia nervosa. Also, owing to the anorexia nervosa and the effect of this condition on a person's physical health, the side effects of the drug treatments may worsen their physical health. If there is no or limited improvement in the person's condition, day care or in-patient care may be required.

Some individuals with anorexia nervosa are so physically unwell due to malnutrition that they need in-patient care immediately. They may have rapid weight loss, and there may be a risk of suicide. Therefore, admission to an in-patient unit is required (Tummey 2005). This may be a specialist eating disorder unit or within an adolescent unit. The focus is on weight gain, carefully monitoring the person's physical condition, but equally psychological treatment should focus on addressing issues of their eating behaviour and their attitudes towards weight and size. Sometimes, a person has to be admitted compulsorily under the Mental Health Act (see Chapter 6 of this book) and fed usually via a nasogastric tube against their will, as their condition is life threatening. This intervention is a last resort.

The carers of the person with anorexia nervosa may feel guilty and upset, wondering what has happened to cause this disorder and trying to establish why they did not identify their child's illness earlier. This is due to the fact that the person is able to conceal their weight loss and their behaviour from everybody, and it is often by accident that their condition is discovered. The carers may also feel anger and resentment, finding it difficult to understand why their child will not eat. Both parents/carers and siblings need to be fully involved in the treatment process of the person with anorexia nervosa and offered support and advice so they can understand the disorder but also in order for them to provide support for their child (Eating Disorders Association 2006b).

Overall, it is important to understand that treatment is a very frightening process for the person with anorexia nervosa. They believe that they had gained control of their lives by gaining control of their dietary intake and so, as that control is being removed from them, the future can now appear very bleak and they may be at risk of attempting suicide. Although their thoughts and behaviour can be difficult to understand (as their lives can be at serious risk due to malnutrition), the health-care practitioner needs to spend time listening to their concerns to understand what precipitated and is perpetuating this disorder. This will demonstrate to the person with anorexia nervosa that the health care professional wishes to elucidate the person's perspective of their illness and will facilitate the development of a therapeutic relationship with them and their family. Therefore, the person can begin to trust the process and participate in the treatment (Tummey 2005).

If untreated, anorexia nervosa has one of highest mortality rates for a mental health disorder, 10–15% of people with anorexia nervosa die from either medical complications or suicide (Semple *et al.* 2005). Of those who receive care and treatment, one-third have a full recovery, one-third have a partial recovery (so they still have some features of the illness) and one-third do not improve at all and have chronic difficulties with food and their weight (Semple *et al.* 2005; Benson & Piero 2004).

Scenario One

Anna is 13 years old. She is the middle child of three siblings. She is intelligent, sensitive and particularly enjoys cooking for her family and friends. She has a caring nature and, like her mother, is described as a 'perfectionist'. Anna has a small circle of very close friends. They all enjoy shopping together for the latest fashions and avidly follow celebrity news and fashion/make-up advice. Recently, they all decided to try a new diet. Initially, they were all very motivated but after a short while they stopped the diet. Anna, however, continued the diet rigidly. She also began an exercise regime consisting of jogging, aerobics and swimming. This regime increased to twice daily. Her friends commented that they rarely saw Anna as she was always busy with all her new exercise activities and when they did meet her she appeared dishevelled, withdrawn and irritable. Her family noticed that, instead of wearing her normal figure-hugging clothes, she was wearing baggy jeans and oversized jumpers.

One day at school, Anna collapsed and her mother was called to accompany her to the hospital where she was shocked to see her daughter's emaciated body and Anna's retort, 'I'm not underweight; I need to lose weight!'

BULIMIA NERVOSA

Symptoms of bulimia nervosa had been discussed as long as medical records have existed; before its definition by the World Health Organization (1992), it was seen as a gastric disorder. One case report of a young woman with bulimia nervosa was published by a Swiss psychiatrist in 1944; however, he had diagnosed schizophrenia. Bulimia nervosa was named by Dr Gerald Russell (a British psychiatrist) in 1979 (Fairburn & Brownell 2002). He reported on 30 patients he had treated who displayed an uncontrolled desire to overeat, practised self-induced vomiting or used laxatives, partook in excessive exercise and had concerns regarding body weight and size. It was termed 'bulimia nervosa' as it was felt to be related to anorexia nervosa (Broussard 2005). A literal translation of 'bulimia nervosa' means 'hunger of an ox'. The term 'bulimia' refers to episodes of uncontrolled eating known as 'binges'. Some people (up to 30%) with anorexia nervosa go on to develop bulimia nervosa (Barker 2003). Similarly to anorexia nervosa, the person may initially be on a diet to lose weight. Unlike anorexia nervosa, the person with bulimia nervosa has normal weight. Therefore, it may be several years before it is evident that the person has features of this disorder. Symptoms of depression are also more common in people with bulimia nervosa (Gelder *et al.* 2001).

Bulimia nervosa usually affects 1–2% of women, usually in their mid-adolescence and early 20s, although bulimia nervosa can present in people up to 40 years old (Semple *et al.* 2005). Unlike anorexia nervosa, people with bulimia nervosa come from a range of social classes, age groups and ethnic backgrounds (Broussard 2005).

Features of bulimia nervosa

For a person to be diagnosed with bulimia nervosa, they usually have the following features:

- persistent preoccupation with eating and irresistable craving for food
- irresistible craving for food
- 'binges' (episodes of overeating) and attempts to counter the effects of food
- morbid fear of fatness with imposed low-weight threshold.

Persistent preoccupation with eating and irresistible craving for food

The person with bulimia nervosa will wish to avoid eating; however, they will be preoccupied with thoughts of food and calorific content. Effectively, they have a profound loss of control over their eating and may refer to themselves as 'failed anorexics' as they are unable to starve themselves (Fairburn & Harrison 2003).

'Binges' and attempts to counter the effects of food

During these episodes, large amounts of food are consumed rapidly, usually foods such as bread, cakes or other sweet foods. This can be very costly and some people with bulimia nervosa are caught shoplifting food. Usually, the person eats alone. After eating, there is initial relief but rapidly this turns into guilt and disgust. These episodes may have been precipitated by a stressful event, sad mood or by deciding to break a period of self-starvation (Eby & Brown 2005). The person is not necessarily hungry but sees food as a comfort.

After the binge eating, the person may then induce vomiting, take laxatives, endure periods of starvation or use drugs (e.g. appetite suppressants) to rid the body of the food in the hope that they will not gain weight. These episodes of binge eating and then purging may occur several times a day (Fontaine 2003).

Louise Roche in her biography *Glutton for Punishment* describes an episode of binge eating:

I close the curtains and sit on the floor surrounded by the food. I turn on the bedside lamp, shut the door and begin to eat. First the toast. I cut thick slices from the still-hard butter and lay them on the toast. I ram piece after piece into my mouth, feeling the butter cold and greasy against the warm, dry toast. I eat piece after piece until it is all gone and then start to eat the chocolate . . . and begin to eat mechanically throwing some pieces to the back of my throat without even tasting them, putting some pieces in slowly and pressing them against the roof of my mouth before scraping them off and pushing them down my throat. (Copyright © Louise Roche, 1984).

Morbid fear of fatness with imposed low-weight threshold

Like the person with anorexia nervosa, the person with bulimia nervosa has a fear of being fat, and they constantly set themselves an unrealistic weight target to achieve. They also have overvalued ideas on what being slim represents and feel if they could reach and maintain their unrealistic ideal weight then life would be much better. They are very self-critical and, like people with anorexia nervosa, are perfectionists in their own standards of behaviour (Fontaine 2003).

Causes of bulimia nervosa

Similar to anorexia nervosa, the person has low self-esteem and is also described as a perfectionist. There is also a personal and/or familial history of obesity. There is generally a familial history of a mental health problem, usually depression. The person with bulimia nervosa will also report a range of adverse childhood experiences such as physical and/or sexual abuse or neglect. They will frequently have endured teasing about their weight and shape from friends and family (Norman & Ryrie 2004).

Care and management of bulimia nervosa

The person with bulimia is usually cared for as an outpatient. Hospital admission only tends to occur if the person has suicidal ideas or physical illnesses or symptoms. Although the person generally is of normal weight, they will require support and understanding by the health care practitioner in order to address their beliefs about eating and their episodes of bingeing.

NICE guidelines for eating disorders (NICE 2004) stipulate that a self-help programme may be the first step. However, instead of this, the person with bulimia nervosa may be prescribed antidepressant therapy, the drug of choice being fluoxetine (Prozac) 60 mg daily (usual dose to treat depression is 20 mg) (Healy 2005). This is because it can reduce the frequency of binge eating and purging. Long-term treatment with medication may be necessary.

Psychological treatments consist of cognitive behavioural therapy (CBT) specifically developed for bulimia nervosa. The person receives between 16 and 20 sessions.

CBT, according to Fairburn and Harrison (2003), has been found to be the most effective treatment for people with bulimia nervosa.

CBT is often split into three phases (Tonks 2003). The first phase consists of learning to reduce bingeing and dieting. The person maintains a diary recording how often they eat, binge and exercise. They are also encouraged to eat small meals throughout the day. Information about bulimia nervosa is also provided by the therapist. During the second phase, they are encouraged to talk more about food, what foods they eat and their feelings about food and weight. During the third phase, Tonks (2003) suggests that the person should be feeling better and with fewer episodes of bingeing and treatment will focus on improving their symptoms further and developing strategies to avoid their symptoms reoccurring. An alternative form of psychological therapy to CBT is interpersonal psychotherapy (as described in the section on anorexia nervosa).

The person experiencing bulimia nervosa will require an understanding and empathic approach to facilitate a discussion of their feelings and behaviour. They feel much shame and embarrassment regarding their binges and subsequent purging and exercise behaviour. Therefore, they will need to see that the health care practitioner will be understanding and supportive before they conceal these symptoms for fear of humiliation and rejection.

Scenario Two

Jane is 21 years old. She is just completing her three years at university, where she is studying fashion and design. She is expected to achieve a first-class honours degree and is concerned that her work will not be good enough to achieve this grade.

She recently became concerned regarding her weight due to comments made to her by her family who said she looked 'just like her father', who is overweight. On confiding with her friend that she felt she had gained weight, her friend agreed with her and recommended a diet. Her sister recently disclosed to Jane that she recalled that both her and Jane were 'touched up' by their uncle (her father's brother).

Jane's diet begins well but she finds it difficult to cope with the overwhelming hunger pangs and thinks about food and the calorific content of food all day. One day, she finds herself in the supermarket filling up a trolley with bread, cakes and sweets that she devours quickly on her own in her student accommodation. After eating all the food she purchased, she feels not only physically sick but has a sense of revulsion about her behaviour. To ease the sense of fullness and to avoid gaining weight, she makes herself vomit. These binges begin to occur more and more frequently, especially when she is at home visiting her family. Jane's mood is noticeably low and eventually after much encouragement she discloses her feelings and behaviour to her sister.

BINGE EATING DISORDER

Binge eating disorder was first seen as a disorder in its own right in 1992. As the name suggests, binge eating disorder is when the person has recurrent episodes of bingeing (as seen in bulimia nervosa) but without the weight control behaviour. The person does not tend to use purgatives, excessive exercise or self-induced vomiting as seen in a person with bulimia nervosa. However, the person with binge eating disorder does experience distress during and after binge eating (Eby & Brown 2005). Usually, the person is obese and tends to be aged between 40 and 50 years old. Approximately one in five of people with binge eating disorder are men. According to Fairburn and Brownell (2002), binge eating disorder affects 2-3% of the population, a much higher percentage is seen in weight-control clinics.

Causes of binge eating disorder

Adverse childhood experiences, tendency to obesity and repeated comments regarding their shape and weight are likely precipitating factors for the development of this disorder (Fairburn & Brownell 2002). This is a relatively new area where there is limited research evidence.

Care and treatment

NICE guidelines (NICE 2004) recommend similar treatments as seen for people with bulimia nervosa. These treatments are a specifically adapted CBT programme for binge eating disorder, interpersonal psychotherapy and antidepressant therapy such as fluoxetine (Prozac). People with this disorder will need similar care and support as those people with bulimia nervosa.

Scenario Three

John, 35 years old, has been referred to see a dietician in his health centre regarding his obesity. He informs the dietician that he has been on a variety of diets to control his weight, but all to no avail. He feels that he is genetically predisposed to obesity as all his family are overweight. The dietician cannot understand why he has not lost weight as he informs her that he hardly eats anything but 'now and again I'll have a feast'. John explains that once to twice a week he can eat up to two loaves of bread with thick butter and jam and a pizza within an hour. He feels ashamed of himself afterwards but feels he cannot control his behaviour. Once he made himself vomit, but this made him feel worse and even more ashamed of himself. He has not discussed his feelings or behaviour with anyone else as he feels so embarrassed.

CONCLUSION

Eating disorders can have a profoundly detrimental effect on a person's physical, psychological and social functioning. All eating disorders have a direct effect on a person's physical health and mortality and in some cases can cause death due to malnutrition or suicide.

It is important to involve the family in all aspects of the person's care (with their consent) so that all the family can understand the causes of the disorder but also to prevent the disorder occurring in one of the other siblings. An understanding and empathic approach facilitating discussion of the person's feelings will enable the person with an eating disorder to begin to trust and work collaboratively with the health care team.

REFERENCES

Barker P (2003) *Psychiatric and Mental Health Nursing: The craft of caring*. London, Hodder Arnold.

Benson NC, Piero (2004) *Introducing Psychiatry*. Cambridge, Icon Books.

Bhugra D, Bhui K, Gupta KR (2000) Bulimic disorders and sociocentric values in north India. *Social Psychiatry and Psychiatric Epidemiology* **35**(2): 86–93.

Braun D, Sunday S, Huang A, Halmi K (1999) More males seek treatment for eating disorders. *International Journal of Eating Disorders* **25**(4): 415–424.

Broussard BB (2005) Women's experiences of bulimia nervosa. *Issues and Innovations in Nursing Practice* **49**(1): 43–50.

Chisholm K (2002) *Hungry Hell: What It's Really Like to Be Anorexic: A Personal Story*. London, Short Books.

Clark-Stone S (2003) Understanding eating disorders. *Nursing Times* **99**(44): 20–26.

Duker M, Slade R (2003) *Anorexia Nervosa & Bulimia: How to Help* (2nd edn.). Buckingham, Open University Press.

Eating Disorders Association (2006a) What is an eating disorder?, http://www.edauk.com/what_is_eating_disorder.htm, accessed 27 April 2006.

Eating Disorders Association (2006b) Caring for someone with an eating disorder, http://www.edauk.com/carers/caring.htm, accessed 27 April 2006.

Eby L, Brown NJ (2005) *Mental Health Nursing Care*, Upper Saddle River, NJ, Pearson/Prentice Hall.

Fairburn CG, Harrison PJ (2003) Eating disorders. *Lancet* **361**(9355): 407–416.

Fairburn CG, Brownell KD (2002) *Eating Disorders and Obesity* (2nd edn.). New York, Guildford Press.

Fontaine K (2003) *Mental Health Nursing* (5th edn.). Upper Saddle River, NJ, Prentice Hall.

Furnham A, Adam-Saib S (2001) Abnormal eating attitudes and behaviours and perceived parental control: a study of white British and British–Asian school girls. *Social Psychiatry and Psychiatric Epidemiology* **36**(9): 462–470.

Gelder M, Mayou R, Cowen P (2001) *Shorter Oxford Textbook of Psychiatry*. Oxford, Oxford University Press.

Healy D (2005) *Psychiatric Drugs Explained*. London, Churchill Livingstone.

Hetherington MM (2000) Eating disorders: diagnosis, etiology and prevention. *Nutrition* **16**(7/8): 547–551.

Kirby SD, Hart DA, Cross D, Mitchell G (eds) (2004) *Mental Health Nursing: Competencies for Practice*. Basingstoke, Palgrave.

Kneisl CR, Wilson HS, Trigoboff E (2004) *Contemporary Psychiatric-Mental Health Nursing*. Upper Saddle River, NJ, Pearson/Prentice Hall.

McClelland L, Crisp A (2001) Anorexia nervosa and social class. *International Journal of Eating Disorders* **29**(2): 150–156.

Murphy B, Manning Y (2003) An introduction to anorexia nervosa and bulimia nervosa. *Nursing Standard* **18**(14–16): 45–52.

National Institute for Health and Clinical Excellence (2004) *Eating Disorders: Core Interventions of Anorexia Nervosa, Bulimia Nervosa, and Related Eating Disorders*. London, National Institute for Health and Clinical Excellence.

Norman I, Ryrie I (2004) *The Art and Science of Mental Health Nursing: A Textbook of Principles and Practice*. Maidenhead, Open University Press.

O'Donnell G (2002) *Mastering Sociology* (4th edn.). Basingstoke, Palgrave.

Paterson A (2004) *Fit to Die: Men and Eating Disorders*. Bristol, Lucky Duck Publishing.

Peate I (2001) Male Eating Disorders. *Practice Nursing* **12**(3): 116–118.

Robinson PH (2000) Review article: recognition and treatment of eating disorders in primary and secondary care. *Alimentary Pharmacology Therapeutics* **14**(4): 367–377.

Roche L (1984) *Glutton for Punishment*. London, Pan Books.

Semple D, Smyth R, Burns J, Darjee R, McIntosh A (2005) *Oxford Textbook of Psychiatry*. Oxford, Oxford University Press.

Tonks A (2003) Information for patients: what happens during cognitive behaviour therapy for bulimia. *British Medical Journal* **327**(7411): 382.

Tummey R (2005) *Planning Care in Mental Health Nursing*. Basingstoke, Palgrave.

World Health Organization (1992) *The ICD-10 Classification of Mental and Behavioural Disorders: Clinical Descriptions and Diagnostic Guidelines*. Geneva, World Health Organization.

10 Dual Diagnosis: Substance Misuse and Mental Health Problems

S. HAHN

INTRODUCTION

The term 'dual diagnosis', or 'comorbidity', refers to the coexistence of a severe mental health problem and substance misuse; however, many people with these experiences describe more than two problems at any one time. This chapter focuses on dual diagnosis because of the way in which each experience may trigger or exacerbate the other. By understanding the relationship between mental health and problematic substance misuse, service providers will be better able to ensure the development of appropriate and effective assessments and interventions. The *Dual Diagnosis Good Practice Guide* (Department of Health 2002) describes four possible relationships between mental health problems and substance misuse:

1. A primary psychiatric illness precipitates or leads to substance misuse.
2. Misuse of substances makes the mental health problem worse or alters its course.
3. Intoxication and/or substance dependence leads to psychological problems.
4. Substance misuse and/or withdrawal leads to psychiatric symptoms or illnesses.

Services get caught up with issues around what is the main problem: which came first, mental health problems or substance misuse? In many ways, this is irrelevant because both may well be a response to emotional and psychological difficulties or trauma. Substance misuse can be a way of coping with problems generally and mental health problems specifically, and to judge those engaging in this behaviour as less deserving of services is unhelpful on one hand and could be described as neglectful on the other.

Other chapters in this book have addressed specific mental health problems, including bipolar disorder, schizophrenia and depression; so these will not be covered here. However, the effects of some drugs will be covered, as will the possible interaction between psychosis, depression and substance misuse be explored.

It is suggested that dual diagnosis is prevalent within mental health and drug and alcohol services, and is increasing. Among CMHTs (community mental health

Caring for Adults with Mental Health Problems   Edited by I. Peate and S. Chelvanayagam
© 2006 John Wiley & Sons, Ltd

teams), 44% of service users report problem drug use and/or harmful alcohol use and 74.5% of clients in treatment for drug problems and 80.6% of those in treatment for alcohol use have had a history of mental health problems within the previous year (Weaver *et al.* 2004). Within the prison service, prevalence of drug dependency and dual diagnosis is high (Department of Health 2002) with 79% of male remand prisoners who are drug dependent having two additional mental health disorders (Hawkins & Gilburt 2004).

Debate and research regarding the cause of dual diagnosis continue and are approached from both angles: 'Why do people with mental health problems use drugs?' and 'What causes mental health problems in people who misuse substances?'

Mental health service users use drugs for the same reasons as other people, namely:

- for pleasure
- to get high
- to relax
- for social interaction.

However, the increase in the misuse of substances in people with mental health problems compared with the general population is not explained by this. Issues such as social exclusion, self-medication and a susceptibility to both conditions have been suggested as possible explanations (Khantzian 1997). There is still uncertainty as to what extent substance misuse can cause mental illness, although there is general agreement that substance misuse may trigger or exacerbate mental illness. Substance misuse may also mask mental illness or, indeed, mimic it. It is important to remember that not only do people react differently to substances depending on when, what and how they are used but also their substance misuse and mental health may vary over time. The experience of dual diagnosis impacts on all areas of the client's life and those around them. People with dual diagnosis experience higher levels of homelessness, victimisation and HIV infection than people with mental illness alone (Drake *et al.* 1991).

The question of 'Which came first?' is often asked as a way of either understanding the problem or, some would suggest, as a way of passing people onto another service. Service users report feeling pushed from service to service.

When you have stopped drinking, you can come to the mental health service.
When your mental health is stable, we will deal with your drug problem.

What service users say is that the relationship between the problems cannot be easily separated and that different service models do not always fit together well. Within mental health services, people are viewed as being ill, and, while encouraged to be independent and to work in partnership with the service providers, are still 'cared for'. In contrast, substance misusers are only perceived to benefit

Table 10.1 Drug classifications (adapted from Drugscope 2006)

Drug	Known as	Type	Classification	Method	Reason for use
Heroin	Smack, Brown, H, Skag, Gear	opiate	A	smoked, injected, oral	relaxation, relief of pain, cold and hunger
Methadone	Green, Script	opiate	A	injected, oral	as for heroin
Cocaine	Coke, Charlie	stimulant	A	sniffed, smoked, injected, oral	energy, confidence, exhilaration, stamina, euphoria
Crack	Rocks, Ice	stimulant	A	smoked	as cocaine
Ecstasy	E, Disco Biscuits	stimulant	A	usually orally, maybe injected or snorted	euphoria, energy then later feeling of empathy and relaxation
LSD	Acid, Trips	hallucinogen	A	orally	well being, hallucinations
Mushrooms	Shrooms, Mushies	hallucinogen	A	orally	as above
Amphetamines	Speed, Whiz, Uppers, Billy	stimulant	B	orally, sniffed, smoked, injected	increased energy and confidence, suppressed appetite
Diazepam	Benzos	depressant	C	swallowed or injected	increase relaxation, reduce anxiety
Temazepam	Tems, Mazzies, Jellies	depressant	C	as above	as above
Anabolic steroids		stimulant	C	tablets or injection	muscle building
Cannabis	Dope, Draw, Resin, Skunk		C	smoked, eaten or drunk	relaxation
Alcohol	Booze, Pop	depressant		drunk	increase confidence, decrease inhibitions

from treatment when they are ready to receive it. Society views these two groups of people differently too. There is generally more compassion and support for people with mental health problems (although there is still stigma and social exclusion), than for substance misusers. People using illegal substances are really expected to take responsibility for their own actions, and any work with the user will only take place when he or she is ready to receive it. Their automatic engagement in illegal behaviour often adds to the problems they experience as a result of their substance misuse (Hawkins & Gilburt 2004).

There has been a lot of research and discussion as to the best way to work with this challenging and often vulnerable group of people (Department of Health 2002), and good-practice guidelines suggest integration and joint working rather than serial or parallel service models (Department of Health 2002). Integrated models of care imply that the same staff provide relevant interventions to meet the mental health and substance-misuse needs of the service users. The staff will be trained and experienced in both fields to enable them to provide a holistic, coordinated service. In the parallel model, treatment and interventions for both conditions are carried out by separate teams, but at the same time. This requires teams to work together and to develop effective liaison. The approach whereby the service user is treated for one condition before accessing services for the other is the serial model.

Further confusion exists because of the legal system and social acceptability. Alcohol use, which causes problems for the greatest number of people, is legal, generally acceptable and often encouraged. It is relatively cheap and easily accessible. Other drugs are categorised under the Misuse of Drugs Act 1971 (Her Majesty's Stationery Office 1971), which reflects how dangerous different drugs are thought to be (Table 10.1). You will notice that prescribed drugs are included in this Act, if they are obtained without a prescription and, if prepared for injection, class B and C drugs become class A.

The impact some drugs may have on mental health is considered below, and, while common types of drugs can have similar effects on mental health, it should be remembered that the effects of any drug will depend on a number of factors (Rasool 2002), including:

- the expectations of the user
- the amount of drug taken
- what other drugs are used
- the individual's existing mental state
- tolerance to the drug
- general physical health.

STIMULANTS

Stimulants (amphetamines, crack, cocaine, ecstasy) can cause or mimic mania, anxiety, depression and paranoid psychosis, and withdrawal can resemble major depression. This cycle may trigger or present as bipolar disorder.

Up to 80% of regular cocaine users experience symptoms of hypomania, which include:

- euphoria
- grandiose ideas
- impaired judgement
- increased psychomotor activity.

In addition, there may be features similar to those seen in schizophrenia, such as visual and auditory hallucinations.

Paranoid feelings may give rise to aggressive behaviour and panic, and continued high doses and long-term use may lead to toxic psychosis with feelings of persecution, loss of insight, hallucinations and delusions. These features usually subside after about 24 hours, but at the time may be indistinguishable from acute psychosis.

Amphetamines can produce similar reactions but, although the psychosis may last longer than that triggered by cocaine, these reactions usually subside within a few days. Psychosis is more likely to occur with long-term use but can be triggered by a single use beginning a day or so afterwards. Features include disordered thinking, hallucinations, delusions, repetitive behaviour and involuntary scratching of the skin (Connell 1958).

HALLUCINOGENS

Hallucinogens (LSD, magic mushrooms) are considered to be unpredictable and to trigger latent mental illness (Hawkins & Gilburt 2004). They may imitate delusions and paranoia associated with psychosis. People who use LSD report flashbacks at a later date as well as panic attacks and physical and psychological exhaustion.

CANNABIS

Cannabis (there is still uncertainty as to what type of drug cannabis is – Drugscope advises that it can be termed both a cannaboid and a hallucinogen) is frequently in the news and the subject of debate in terms of the relationship between its use and mental illness. Its use is more widely acceptable socially and, in 2002, it was reclassified as a class C from a class B drug. Cannabis is the most commonly used illegal substance.

Cannabis is generally regarded as a depressant but can have both hallucinatory and stimulant effects (Hawkins & Gilburt 2004). Debate continues as to the role of cannabis in triggering or causing mental illness. High doses and continued use can lead to a toxic confusional state and acute psychotic reactions that are difficult to distinguish from schizophrenic-type psychosis can also occur. Other features associated with mental illness include:

- lethargy
- panic attacks
- paranoia
- short-term memory loss
- demotivation.

The term 'amotivational syndrome' was devised to describe a cluster of features associated with regular cannabis use, including:

- apathy
- loss of ambition
- impaired concentration
- deterioration in academic performance.

Together, these features present as personality change, but are more likely a result of chronic intoxication.

The relationship between cannabis and mental health relates to the strength of the drug, the frequency of use and the age at which people begin using it (Iverson 2004). Cannabis is a drug of dependence and the risks associated with mental illness are increased the earlier young people start using it. It has also been suggested that cannabis dependence has a role in predicting increased risk of using other illicit drugs. Research continues into the causal links between cannabis and mental illness, and evidence is growing to support the belief that cannabis can be a contributory cause of psychotic symptoms (Hall 2006). Studies that support links between cannabis use and developing schizophrenia acknowledge an existing predisposition to the latter (Smit et al 2004).

The prevalence and nature of cannabis use amongst those with severe mental health problems in community-based services in an inner-city area of the UK was assessed; 43% of the clients were misusing cannabis (Graham & Maslin 2002). Within mental health services, cannabis, second to alcohol, was the substance most commonly used problematically. Problematic cannabis use was most frequently associated with males and a diagnosis of schizophrenia, schizotypal or delusional disorders. 'Pleasure enhancement' and 'coping' were most commonly given as the reasons for use.

OPIATES

This group of drugs (heroin, methadone) is used for the relief of physical and psychological pain and may mask presenting psychiatric features, which might emerge when use of the drug is reduced or stopped. There are physical problems associated with injecting, and difficulties relating to accessing the drug and dependence.

DEPRESSANTS (ALCOHOL, BENZODIAZEPINES)

Alcohol consumption is generally accepted and openly advertised in many Western countries. This social acceptability has been blamed in part for the high rates of dependence. Countries where alcohol is more available have higher rates of alcoholism (Action on Addiction 2006). Alcohol is a depressant, although people experience increased confidence and may be more sociable due to lowered inhibitions.

Links between alcohol abuse and suicide, both attempted and completed, are well documented (Sher 2006). People misusing alcohol may develop the following features of mental illness:

- low mood
- agitation
- apathy
- loss of appetite
- loss of libido
- suicidal ideation.

The depressant effect of alcohol may contribute to suicidal thoughts, and impulsivity and aggression are strongly implicated in suicidal behaviour and also common to people intoxicated by alcohol.

Intoxicated people are more likely to attempt suicide using more lethal methods, and alcohol may be important in suicides among individuals with no previous psychiatric history (Department of Health 2003).

Alcohol misuse can also result in vitamin B1 deficiency, which may lead to Wernike's encephalopathy (features of this are confusion, staggering gait and abnormal eye movements). This can lead to Korsakoff's syndrome if not treated, which is characterised by severe memory impairment, confabulation and lack of insight (Alzheimer's Society 2006).

Chronic misuse of alcohol may result in alcoholic hallucinosis, which may be difficult to distinguish from schizophrenia. Persecutory auditory hallucinations may occur in clear consciousness, and may appear during periods of abstinence, reduction or continued use.

BENZODIAZEPINES

This group of drugs includes diazepam, temazepam, nitrazepam, all of which are prescribed drugs. If these drugs are obtained without a prescription, they come under class B of the Misuse of Drugs Act 1971, and if prepared for injection are classed as class A drugs.

Benzodiazepines are depressants and prescribed to treat symptoms of anxiety and sleeping difficulties. Guidelines are that they should only be prescribed for short-term use as they are addictive (British Medical Association/Royal Pharmaceutical Society 2006), and should not be prescribed to people with a history of drug or alcohol dependence. Some people become aggressive, hostile, agitated and experience perceptual disorders when using benzodiazepines. Abrupt withdrawal may result in confusion, toxic psychosis and convulsions. This demonstrates how features common to mental illness can result from both misuse and withdrawal of these drugs (Hawkins & Gilburt 2004).

SUBSTANCE MISUSE IN PEOPLE WITH PSYCHIATRIC DISORDERS

Having described the possible impact of some commonly misused drugs on mental health, it may be useful to approach the situation from the perspective of substance misuse in people with diagnosed psychiatric disorders.

Studies show that up to 50% of people with schizophrenia have either a drug or alcohol problem (Menezes *et al.* 1996). Both conditions feature the impairment of social functioning, cognitive ability, emotional state and relationships; so it is understandable that, when combined, the impact of both conditions compounds any initial symptoms or features. Substance misuse may worsen existing psychotic features of schizophrenia, such as hallucinations, delusions and lack of insight, or the same individual may experience these features as a direct consequence of their substance misuse. The resulting experience will depend on the type and strength of the drug used.

Cocaine, cannabis and alcohol have been noted to exacerbate existing psychotic symptoms and to affect treatment of the condition. Service users report things differently. They report using non-prescribed drugs to alleviate boredom, help to socialise, relieve anxiety and depression, help with sleep or to cope with the side effects of prescribed medication (Mueser *et al.* 1998).

The effects of non-prescribed drugs tend to be short lived, and the service user then has to cope with any experience of withdrawal and activity associated with getting and paying for the drugs. Mental health service users are then engaged in illegal activity and vulnerable to arrest and involvement with the criminal justice system.

Substance misuse is recognised to be detrimental to the long-term outcome and prognosis of schizophrenia. Working effectively with this group of people presents challenges to service delivery and attitudes to substance misuse. There is often discrepancy between what the service and the service user see as a priority in terms of which of the service user's needs should be addressed first. Only by understanding the service user's experience of their life can staff engage and begin the process of intervention (Barber 2002).

ANXIETY DISORDER

Studies have shown considerable links between anxiety disorders and substance misuse, particularly alcohol, in terms of triggering feelings of anxiety but also as a form of self-medication (Lingford-Hughes 2002). People with anxiety disorders may use alcohol or drugs to cope with their symptoms; however, alcohol and drug misuse may result in anxiety disorder. Links have also been shown between living with people with anxiety disorder and use of alcohol among family members.

MOOD DISORDERS

The relationship between substance misuse and mood disorders is a complex one. There is no doubt that the effect drugs have can depend on the mood the person is in before using them and the expectation they have of the outcome. Mood changes are also affected by the type of drug, its strength, frequency of use and withdrawal. Again, individuals with a mood disorder may use substances to self-medicate in order to achieve some relief from their symptoms. A significant number of people admitted to hospital for a first episode of bipolar disorder had been misusing alcohol for the year preceding their admission, and this type of history often leads to a poorer outcome for the individual (Sonne & Brady 2002).

Substance misuse should be routinely considered when assessing people with mood disorders. It has been suggested that alcohol misuse and depression may well be different expressions of the same underlying cause, depending on gender.

Men have a higher incidence of alcoholism and secondary depression, whereas more women develop alcohol problems following depression. Effective treatment for mood disorders has been demonstrated to have a positive impact on alcohol dependence, but there is less evidence to show that the treatment of mood symptoms results in a reduction of the misuse of other drugs.

By understanding what benefits the service user gets from their non prescribed drug misuse, practitioners may be able to suggest alternatives, which include cognitive behavioural approaches, changing prescribed medication and helping detoxification.

CHILDREN

The existence of dual diagnosis often results in problems associated with housing, relationships, finances and the criminal justice system. There are also considerable issues in relation to parental substance misuse and its effect on the children of drug misusers.

Children and families generally are affected by dual diagnosis. Unpredictability, involvement with different services and poor treatment outcomes commonly associated with this group of people can have an impact on relationships within and the well-being of family members. By being parented by dually diagnosed service users, children are vulnerable to losing a parent through death or by being placed into foster care. In the UK, approximately 300,000 children are adversely affected by drug misuse and 800,000 by alcohol abuse (Advisory Council 2003).

The effects on children range from missed schooling, increased risk of sexual, physical and emotional abuse, anxiety, social exclusion, poverty and of them becoming users.

The impact on the mental health of children has been well documented and those exposed to cocaine use show higher levels of Attention Deficit Hyperactivity Disorder and defiant behaviour by the age of six years (Linares *et al.* 2006).

ASSESSMENT AND TREATMENT APPROACHES

Substance misuse among people with mental health problems is recognised as being usual rather than exceptional; so it follows that mental health services should consider it routinely in assessment and be prepared to offer appropriate treatment and intervention. Adopting a comprehensive and inclusive assessment approach will lead to clearer diagnosis, treatment and information. The way substance misuse is perceived as deviant often results in the mental health service user being reluctant to discuss the extent of their drug use. If service users believe they will either be refused treatment or referred on, they are less likely to engage with the services, resulting in poor treatment outcomes (Hawkins & Gilburt 2004). Assessment should include risks associated with substance misuse and mental health problems and should be part of holistic treatment plans.

There are a number of differences in the approaches of mental health and drug services, which are reinforced by rigid professional boundaries and the lack of staff training. Attitudes and policies that discriminate against service users should be challenged. Kingston CDAT (Community Drug and Alcohol Team) has moved away from a 'no motivation – no service' approach common to substance misuse agencies, and a number of mental health services have moved from their position of being unable, or unwilling, to offer a service unless people are free of non-prescribed substances. These changes are more likely to take place when staff understand the links between mental health problems and substance misuse. Failure to recognise these links results in service users not getting appropriate services and staff becoming increasingly disillusioned and burnt out (Department of Health 2002).

Joint training and working across boundaries are possible ways forward; if services can work together, they are more likely to engage with service users, establish effective interventions and reduce duplication of work. Mainstream mental health services have a responsibility to meet the needs of people with dual diagnosis (Department of Health 2002). To do this effectively, staff need appropriate training and to develop links with specialist substance misuse agencies.

Both substance misuse and severe mental illness are often long-term conditions whereby the client may have periods of stability and relapse; so practitioners should adopt a positive and optimistic approach and consider treatment as an ongoing process. This can be difficult, as working with this group of people is recognised as being extremely challenging. Good and regular supervision is required and caseloads should be monitored and kept at a realistically workable level.

The Department of Health (2002) highlights four stages of treatment, which are:

- engagement
- motivation for change

- active treatment
- relapse prevention.

Engagement refers to establishing and maintaining a therapeutic alliance between the service user and agency staff and is best achieved by developing a non-confrontational and empathic approach to the individual's substance misuse. By addressing their immediate needs, such as health, financial, housing, rather than primarily seeking ways to get a service user to stop misusing substances, the health professional is less likely to make the service user feel threatened and judged, which will make for a better therapeutic alliance.

Establishing the service user's motivation for change is important. This can be achieved by exploring their perspective and the benefits they get from using substances. Recognising that there are positive benefits for their substance misuse will enable the practitioner to explore possible alternatives. For instance, if the service user smokes cannabis to help them sleep, perhaps alternatives could be suggested, such as reducing the use of stimulants, exploring expectations associated with sleep or prescribing medication, and lifestyle changes should also be explored.

Considering their current and past problems and the influence substance misuse had on them may encourage the service user to be motivated towards change. Setting out lists of pros and cons associated with the drug and giving clear, accurate information about the effect of the drug on their mental health may also be beneficial (Derricott *et al.* 1999).

It is essential, though, that information is given in a factual way and not to coerce or attempt to frighten the service user to change; rather they should be invited to consider the information given to them. Service users report feeling that mental health workers often fail to ask why clients misuse substances; instead they report that mental health workers use terms such as 'non-compliance', which carries a negative and sabotaging connotation (Miller & Rollnick 1991).

These techniques are elements of 'motivational interviewing' (Miller & Rollnick 1991), an intervention considered to be effective when working with substance misusers. It is based on the idea that for any change to take place the substance misuser needs to be motivated, and in order to get to this point they will need to see how reducing their substance misuse will improve their mental health and life generally.

Recognising that it may take months for a service user to be ready to change their substance misuse suggests staff need to be patient and develop ways of staying engaged and not disillusioned. At the same time, the substance misusers may still require support to manage their mental health problems.

Ways forward to establishing effective intervention strategies begin with better integration between services and clear working protocols. Exploring attitudes, challenging stereotypes and improving communication are the first steps to developing better relationships across services (Department of Health 2002).

Mapping existing services in an area will provide information as to what is available and how best to move forward. Following exploration of established agencies and their role within dual diagnosis, discussion can take place as to the options available to service users. Developing care pathways, service aims and perceived roles within dual diagnosis will help to clarify gaps in existing provision and areas for development. It is necessary to be clear about the service model to be used. Treatment interventions may include but are not limited to:

- joint treatment approaches
- assertive outreach
- motivational interventions
- individual counselling
- social support
- long-term plans.

Relapse prevention should be part of the ongoing process. Encouraging service users to consider how they will manage relapse and to recognise triggers for relapse will empower them and facilitate a sense of responsibility and control over their experience. Staff will need to be flexible and avoid being punitive or critical of relapses.

Current guidelines encourage harm-reduction techniques in preference to purely abstinence-based programmes (Department of Health 2002). However, this does not mean if abstinence is the service user's aim that it should not be considered, but done so using a step-by-step approach, and by setting realistic, attainable goals.

Attention needs to be paid to service users' social networks and meaningful activities. Having little to do in the day apart from mixing with other people who misuse substances adds to the difficulty people experience in changing their lives. Re-establishing family contacts helps many people, and developing a sense of self-esteem has been found to be effective in helping people to move on.

Low self-esteem develops from 'a learned, negative global judgement about self which shapes how a person thinks, feels and acts on a day to day basis' (Fennell 1999). Increased self-esteem has been found to act as a protective factor against depression, suicidal behaviour and substance misuse, and low self-esteem is common in dual diagnosis (Lecomte *et al.* 1999).

CONCLUSION

This chapter has set out to explain the possible links between substance misuse and mental illness. The difficulties in determining which comes first presents continuing challenges to practitioners; however, the important thing is to work with the individual and their presenting experience. This can be best achieved in the context of a therapeutic and non-judgemental relationship.

Agencies need to establish effective working relationships and policies to ensure service users' needs are met, and the need for appropriate training must be recognised. Staff training should include aspects of mental health and substance misuse, and as the *Good Practice Guide* (Department of Health 2002) encourages, mental health services should take responsibility for this group of people and develop outreach services that recognise the need for supportive, inclusive services.

Where integrated services are not established, the aim should be to ensure parallel rather than serial service provision, as the latter has the poorest outcome.

While people with mental health problems face stigma and social exclusion, those with substance misuse problems face the added stigmas associated with perceptions that their problems are self-inflicted, that their behaviour is antisocial, often immoral and frequently involves criminal actions. So people with both diagnoses have a lot to contend with. It is important to recognise and assess risk relating to the service user and their families, particularly when there are children involved (Howe 2005). Given the increased risk of suicide among people with dual diagnosis, all assessments should explore and record previous attempts and current thoughts of suicide (Department of Health 2002).

Developing strategies that include motivational approaches with those of care will offer dual-diagnosed service users support and understanding of the effect substance misuse has on their mental health. Information and the opportunity to explore their behaviour and the motivation behind it is empowering and may lead to the individual making positive lifestyle changes (Miller & Rollnick 1991).

The causes of substance abuse and mental health problems are complex and involve social, environmental, biological and genetic factors. The service user should be offered treatment to meet their personal needs in terms of the presenting features and underlying causes of their personal experience.

REFERENCES

Action on Addiction (2006) Causes of addiction, http://www.aona.co.uk/addiction/alcohol/causes-of-addiction, accessed 20 July 2006.

Advisory Council (2003) Hidden harm?, http://www.drugs.gov.uk/publication-search/acmd/hidden-harm?view=Binary, accessed 20 July 2006.

Alzheimer's Society (2006) Factsheets, http://www.alzheimers.org.uk/Facts_about_dementia/What_is_dementia/info_Korsakoffs.htm, accessed 20 July 2006.

Barber JG (2002) *Social Work with Addictions* (2nd edn.). Basingstoke, Palgrave Macmillan.

British Medical Association and Royal Pharmaceutical Society of Great Britain (2006) *British National Formulary*. London, British Medical Association and Royal Pharmaceutical Society of Great Britain.

Connell PH (1958) *Amphetamine Psychosis: Institute of Psychiatry Maudsley Monographs Number 5*. London, Oxford University Press.

Department of Health (2002) *Mental Health Policy Implementation Guide. Dual Diagnosis Good Practice Guide*. London, The Stationery Office.

Department of Health (2003) *Health of the Nation Key Areas Handbook: Mental Health*. London, The Stationery Office.

Derricott J, Preston A, Hunt N, Speed S (1999) *The Safer Injecting Briefing*. Liverpool, HIT.

Drake RE, Osher FC, Wallach MA (1991) Homelessness and dual diagnosis. *American Psychologist* **46**(11): 1149–1158.

Drugscope (2006) Drug search, http://www.drugscope.org.uk/druginfo/drugsearch/home2.asp, accessed 20 July 2006.

Fennell M (1999) Low self-esteem. In Tarrier N, Wells A, Haddock G (eds) *Treating Complex Cases*. Chichester, Wiley, pp. 57–73.

Graham HL, Maslin J (2002) Problematic cannabis use amongst those with severe mental health problems in an inner city area of the UK. *Quaternay* **27**(2): 261–273.

Hall W (2006) Cannabis use and the mental health of young people. *Australian and New Zealand Journal of Psychiatry*. **40**(2): 105–113.

Hawkins C, Gilburt H (2004) *Dual Diagnosis Toolkit. Mental health and substance misuse*. London, Rethink/Turning Point.

Her Majesty's Stationery Office (1971) Misuse of Drugs Act 1971, http://www.drugs.gov.uk/drugs-laws/misuse-of-drugs-act/, accessed 20 July 2006.

Howe D (2005) *Child Abuse and Neglect, Attachment, Development and Intervention*. Basingstoke, Palgrave Macmillan.

Iverson L (2004) 'Cannabis and psychiatric illness'. Paper presented at the Cannabis and Mental Health Conference, 20 April 2004, London.

Khantzian EJ (1997) The self-medication hypothesis of addictive disorders: a reconsideration and recent applications. *Harvard Review of Psychiatry* **4**(5): 231–244.

Lecomte T, Cyr M, Lesage AD, Wilde J, Leclerc C, Ricard N (1999) Efficacy of self esteem: module in the empowerment of individuals with schizophrenia. *Journal of Nervous and Mental Disorders* **187**(7): 406–413.

Linares T, Singer LT, Kirchner H, Short EJ, Min MO, Hussey P, Minnes S (2006) Mental health outcomes of cocaine-exposed children at 6 years of age. *Journal of Pediatric Psychology* **31**(1): 85–97.

Lingford-Hughes A, Potokar J, Nutt D (2002) Treating anxiety complicated by substance misuse. *Advances in Psychiatric Treatment* **8**: 107–116.

Menezes PR, Johnson S, Thornicroft G, Marshall J, Prosser D, Bebbington P, Kuipers E Drug and alcohol problems among individuals with severe mental illness in south London. *British Journal of Psychiatry* **168**(5): 612–619.

Miller W, Rollnick S (1991) *Motivational Interviewing: Preparing People to Change Addictive Behaviour*. New York, Guildford Press.

Mueser KT, Drake RE, Wallach MA (1998) Dual diagnosis: a review of etiological theories. *Addictive Behaviors* **23**(6): 717–734.

Rasool GH (2002) *Dual Diagnosis: Substance Misuse and Psychiatric Disorders*. Oxford, Blackwell Science.

Sher L (2006) Alcohol and suicide: neurobiological and clinical aspects. *Scientific World Journal* **6**: 700–706.

Smit F, Boiler L, Cuijpers P (2004) Cannabis use and the risk of later schizophrenia: a review. *Addiction* **99**(4): 425–430.

Sonne SC, Brady KT (2002) Bi-polar disorders and alcoholism. *Alcohol Research and Health* **26**(2): 103–108.

Weaver T, Stimson G, Tyrer P, Barnes T, Renton A (2004) What are the implications for clinical management and service development of prevalent comorbidity in UK mental health and substance misuse treatment populations? *Drugs: Education, Prevention and Policy* **11**(4): 329–348.

11 Schizophrenia and Schizophrenia-type Disorders

Y. MITCHELL

INTRODUCTION

This chapter aims to inform the reader about, and dispel the myths surrounding this enduring and rather tenacious of all mental illness. 'Schizophrenia' is a term that can fill some members of the public with fear and anxiety. The very diagnosis is self-isolating, and people who do not understand this particular illness may avoid those who display rather unpleasant and sometimes dramatic symptoms. The impact of schizophrenia on the person and their family will also be addressed as well as the ways in which service users and carers can be involved in programmes of rehabilitation. Current treatment options will be considered by addressing the role of those who provide mental health strategies – the multidisciplinary team – whose therapeutic relationships with the service user are vital to that person's sense of control.

A person with schizophrenia experiences periods of psychosis. 'Psychosis' refers to the mental state of experiencing reality in a different way from others. People who experience psychosis assume that others perceive the world as they do, and they become puzzled as to why others are not reacting in a similar manner. The overall goal is to facilitate recognition of psychotic features and help to develop coping strategies to manage symptoms. These symptoms manifest through a complicated neurobiological brain disease, affecting the person's ability to process information. The behaviours associated with these disruptions are difficult to understand. They are usually persistent and severe in nature and can have a damaging effect on the person's life.

The person with schizophrenia is usually frightened by these experiences and has great difficulty forming and sustaining relationships, particularly meeting new people. They become severely disabled and tend to be alienated from society (Eby & Brown 2005). There are varying degrees of psychotic features in other forms of mental illness, for example puerperal psychosis following the birth of a child, a woman may develop false beliefs (delusional) in which she may think that the baby is the devil. Another form is bipolar disorder, which ranges from periods of depression to elation with psychotic features.

Caring for Adults with Mental Health Problems Edited by I. Peate and S. Chelvanayagam
© 2006 John Wiley & Sons, Ltd

Catatonia is a rare form of psychotic behaviour, often associated with schizophrenia and the psychomotor behaviour of movement and walking. The ability to pick up objects, for example, is severely impaired. In its most profound form, a person suffering from catatonia could display either severe agitation or restlessness to the extreme of almost a statuesque presentation and their body could be witnessed as coming to a standstill. This behaviour appears to be completely out of the person's control and can be maintained for long periods of time (Kneisl *et al.* 2004). Eating and drinking can be very difficult to sustain and carers may face challenges when administering fluids, medication, diet and all forms of activities of living. Catatonia is rare, dramatic and startling, particularly for families and carers to witness. Treatment programmes are based on gently and slowly engaging with the person and encouraging them back to reality.

SCHIZOAFFECTIVE DISORDER

With this disorder, people experience a combination of psychotic features such as delusions, hallucinations and disorganised behaviour but will also have features of a mood disorder such as depression and/or mania (hyperactivity); this disorder is more common in women (Fontaine 2003). Therefore, someone with this disorder may have previously been diagnosed with either schizophrenia or a mood disorder such as bipolar disorder.

BRIEF PSYCHOTIC EPISODE

There is a rapid onset of this condition that may be precipitated by a stressful event. The person will present with features of a thought disorder with delusions and hallucinations, and usually all these features resolve within a month. The person experiencing a brief psychotic disorder may require short-term admission to an acute mental health admission unit and treatment with antipsychotic medication (Semple *et al.* 2005). This chapter focuses on the most profound and persistent form of psychosis: schizophrenia.

Schizophrenia, is a combination of two Greek words: *schizein* 'to split' and *phren* 'mind'. However, the Swiss psychiatrist Eugene Bleuler was the first to introduce the term 'schizophrenia', in 1911, believing that this was not a split of personality, referring to two separate identities, that the separation, or split-ting, referred to the cognitive, or thinking, component and the emotional aspects which had separated or split from one another (Donnellan 2000). As a diag-nosis, schizophrenia is demoralising and stigmatising, affecting one in 100 of the general population (Stuart & Laraia 2005). Schizophrenia affects men and women equally, although the age of onset tends to be earlier in men (Gelder *et al.* 2001).

The majority of people develop the illness in adolescence or early adulthood, only 10–15% develop this disorder over the age of 45 (Fontaine 2003). The incidence of schizophrenia are:

- 15–20% of people with schizophrenia fully recover after their first episode and do not suffer subsequent episodes.
- The majority of people with schizophrenia have periods of good health with occasional problems (Donnellan 2000).
- 55% of people with schizophrenia show good to fair social functioning when assessed 13 years after their first episode of schizophrenia (Semple *et al.* 2005).

Ten per cent of people diagnosed with schizophrenia commit suicide usually within the first year of being diagnosed with the condition (Gelder *et al.* 2001). Furthermore, people with schizophrenia can lead unhealthy lifestyles and develop disordered eating patterns, which may mean they are at risk of developing diabetes, heart disease or stroke (cerebrovascular accident); and as a result their mortality rates can be 1.5 times higher than the rest of the population (Jones 2004).

FEATURES OF SCHIZOPHRENIA

Diagnosed by the presence of particular symptoms, schizophrenia commonly falls within two main groups of both positive and negative behaviour. These unusual behaviours, positive features in this case, indicate that they are definite or dominant and are rather peculiar. These positive symptoms refer to the more pronounced or unusual behaviour that strays remarkably from the norm, for example hallucinations (seeing things that are not seen by other people, or hearing voices that may be of a pleasant or unpleasant content).

Negative symptoms refer usually to the deconstruction of normal everyday behaviour, for example slowly withdrawing from social events which then becomes an acute form of social isolation or losing one's motivational drive and direction in life. A person with schizophrenia may demonstrate an alteration in their speech pattern, for example there may be either an absence or poverty of speech as the person seems to speak in a very limited and notably different way, with some new words that others will not recognise. These words are known as neologisms (new, unfamiliar words) and terms such as 'word salads' are used to describe these (Thomson & Mathias 2003). These are a confusing mixture of words, usually meaningless in their context. As it becomes difficult to correct another adult, or question them on their presentation, non health care professionals and families fear for the new and different person before them, as they become more unpredictable in their behaviour. Eventually, the person perceives their differences and feels safer alone, preferring their own company. Mistrust appears to go alongside their need to be remote and distant from other people. The person does not have the same need to talk to anyone, as they rely more on themselves and may leave home only to buy groceries and return. These symptoms are usually present for at least one month or more before diagnosis and either two or more of the positive or negative symptoms present (World Health Organization 1992). The features of schizophrenia affect a person's thoughts, behaviour, mood (affect) and perception, and these will now be defined and described in detail.

THOUGHTS

The person with schizophrenia may experience impairment in their thoughts, memory, language and concentration. They usually experience delusions, which are fixed, false beliefs. The delusions can be delusions of grandeur, such as the person believing they are the King of England (this is seen more commonly in bipolar disorder), or they may be persecutory, in that someone is trying to harm them, for example the person believes that the police are going to kill them (Kneisl *et al.* 2004). (See Scenario One.)

Scenario One: Delusions and false beliefs

Brian thought he was putting on a great deal of weight. As he had always been thin, he was not used to this. He had been taking Stelazine (trifluoperazine), an antipsychotic medication. This weight gain was so unusual that he thought he just must be pregnant. It prayed on his mind and eventually he cut through his stomach with the outer case of a Biro pen he had found to be absolutely sure that he was not pregnant. He eventually told his sister about this and she wept for the man and brother before her. At that time, he told her he knew that it was a strange thing to do, but he also could not help himself from checking to make absolutely certain.

The person with schizophrenia may also describe what is called 'passivity phenomena'. This means that they feel their thoughts and behaviours are controlled by someone or something else.

Ideas of reference are that the person with schizophrenia attributes the actions and speech content of others as having direct reference to them (Barker 2003). Therefore, they may be seen approaching someone on public transport and commenting on their conversation stating, 'I know that you're trying to tell me to start working for the police.' This is a very frightening and bewildering experience for both the person with schizophrenia and the person at whom this is directed.

The person with schizophrenia may also experience 'thought broadcasting'. This is the belief that their thoughts can be heard by others. For example, an adolescent schoolboy may believe that all his school friends know that he is fond of a certain teacher even though he has not told them. 'Thought insertion' may also be experienced by the person with schizophrenia, where they believe that thoughts have been inserted into their brain by something or somebody else, or conversely 'thought withdrawal', where the service user with schizophrenia believes their thoughts can be removed by someone or something else. Poverty of thought may also be experienced, where the service user with schizophrenia reports that they have no thoughts.

One type of thought disorder can be observed by the health care professional and this is 'thought blocking'. The service user will suddenly stop talking as if they have been interrupted. This can occur several times during a conversation (Fontaine 2003).

A person with schizophrenia will also have difficulty maintaining a flow of conversation as their thinking is disorganised and their ideas may move inappropriately from one topic to another. This is known as 'knight's move thinking', as in a knight's L-shaped move during a game of chess, which appears to be illogical. The person may also use 'clang association' when speaking. This means that two words that sound the same but with a different meaning are linked together in a conversation, for example the *sun* is shining and your *son* is unwell. (Gelder *et al.* 2001).

It can also be noted that the person will focus on facts and details and think in a very concrete manner; this is known as 'concrete thinking'. An example of this would be when asked, 'How did you sleep last night?' the person with schizophrenia would reply, 'In a bed.'

Memory impairments and difficulty concentrating due to thought disorder (as described above) will be demonstrated. This will understandably cause the service user difficulties in absorbing and retaining information. It also has been discovered that people diagnosed with schizophrenia have memory and cognitive deficits that precede the onset of schizophrenia (Semple *et al.* 2005).

BEHAVIOUR

The person with schizophrenia may exhibit bizarre behaviour (see Scenario Two). They may present as hyperactive and unpredictable. Bizarre behaviour may consist of the repetition of certain gestures or postures, such as skipping or standing facing a wall. Some people with schizophrenia will copy other people's behaviours, which is known as 'echopraxia', or copy their speech which is known as 'echolalia'. Negative signs include a lack of motivation, self-neglect and decreased activity; a person may lie in bed all day and not get up even to attend to personal hygiene (Kneisl *et al.* 2004).

Scenario Two: Bizarre behaviour

Brian thought he had invented an ideal structure to eradicate stress for ever. It was a good invention. It comprised a mini-Stonehenge and some paper. You place all your thoughts in code on pieces of paper, then tear them into smaller pieces. Then you 'place them into the centre of the model and burn them slowly; it would help to clear your mind'. He wrote to solicitors to patent his ideas, before someone else would get their hands on them. He believed it would help many people deal with their stress and thought he could become quite wealthy if his invention took off.

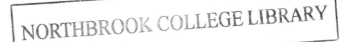

MOOD (AFFECT)

The person with schizophrenia may demonstrate what is known as 'incongruity of affect'; this means that their response to certain conversations or situations would be inappropriate. For example, when they are informed that their dog has died they may laugh aloud, showing a lack of sensitivity. The health care professional may also observe a 'blunted affect', which means that although they state they feel happy this is not demonstrated by smiling or laughter, but instead they appear very stilted. This should not be confused with 'anhedonia'. This is defined as an inability to experience pleasure, particularly in activities that were previously enjoyed (Eby & Brown 2005). Therefore, the world can appear a very frightening and depressing place for the person with schizophrenia as they have difficulties interacting with others and may have little or no enjoyment in their lives.

PERCEPTION

The person with schizophrenia will experience hallucinations. A 'hallucination' is a false perception that can affect any five of the senses. The most common hallucinations are auditory hallucinations, affecting 50–80% of people with schizophrenia (Fontaine 2003). Auditory hallucinations are frequently persecutory, saying negative comments to the person or providing a running commentary on their behaviour. They may also provide the person with commands which can mean that the person's behaviour becomes unpredictable as they are compelled to act on these commands, which may include harm to others or themselves.

Visual hallucinations usually consist of seeing a clearly defined object and are the second-most-common type of hallucination in schizophrenia (Fontaine 2003). Sometimes, a person with schizophrenia can be observed responding to the voices by shouting at them to stop and they can become very frightened. They may be reluctant to inform health care practitioners as they are fearful of the consequences but with support and encouragement may inform their carers (Sims 1995).

SOCIAL AND OCCUPATIONAL DYSFUNCTION

Other prominent features of schizophrenia are the effects on a person's social and occupational functioning. The onset of schizophrenia is usually very slow (insidious), with small changes to personal circumstances, beginning with a gradual withdrawal from peers and friends. In a young person, it may be precipitated by a family event or crisis, for example divorce, leaving home or examination pressure at school or university.

The first symptoms could be viewed initially as a form of shyness, which becomes more pronounced to that of self-isolation or staying in bed during the day and rising at night when others are asleep. Families report changes in routine where the person stops joining them for meals and eats alone in their room. These symptoms impact on the person's relationship with their family. Ultimately, social connections become disconnected and they fail to return calls to friends. Subsequently, their friends, especially young people, who have their own social pursuits in adolescence gradually drift away. It is understandable that problems in sustaining and forming new interpersonal and close relationships become more difficult. A younger person may have experienced employment; however, when a person is so debilitated at home they are very unlikely to secure or maintain their position (Social Exclusion Unit 2004).

CAUSES OF SCHIZOPHRENIA

There are a range of concepts regarding the causes of schizophrenia and much research, for example studies of twins, has been completed to try and establish the main causes. Below are some of the main theories regarding the causes of schizophrenia.

GENETIC FACTORS

Schizophrenia is more likely to occur in a family with a person with schizophrenia. If a sibling has been diagnosed with schizophrenia, there is an 8% risk for another sibling to experience schizophrenia. If one parent has schizophrenia, there is a 13% risk; if both parents have schizophrenia, there is a 40% risk that a child will experience the disorder (Fontaine 2003). However, this evidence is not strong enough to suggest that schizophrenia is a genetic disorder but only that genetics may play a part in the development of the disorder (Eby & Brown 2005).

BIOLOGICAL FACTORS

Eby and Brown (2005) state that there are differences in the structural, chemical and functional aspects of the brains of people with schizophrenia. One particular idea that supports the use of antipsychotic medications is that people with schizophrenia have an excess of the brain chemical dopamine which can be reduced with antipsychotic medication by blocking the neurotransmitter that produces it. This is why some people taking antipsychotic medication experience stiffness, lack of movement or abnormal movements similar to those seen in Parkinson's disease, as Parkinson's disease is caused by a reduction of dopamine in the brain (Healy 2005).

ENVIRONMENTAL FACTORS

Semple *et al.* (2005) report that complications during the mother's pregnancy and a subsequent traumatic delivery of the baby who endures injury have been found to be associated with a risk of developing schizophrenia. Eby and Brown (2005) suggest that people with schizophrenia tend to be born in winter and spring. This has led to a belief that the mother of the person with schizophrenia contracted a maternal viral infection (influenza) that may have affected the infant.

This may link to the fact that most people raised in an urban area have a greater risk for developing the disorder as viral infection is more prevalent in urban areas, (Eby & Brown 2005).

PSYCHOLOGICAL FACTORS

In the late 1950s, Brown (1959) discovered that people with schizophrenia discharged from a psychiatric hospital to live with their family or a relative were more likely to suffer a relapse in their condition than those who were discharged to live alone or without family members. This led to a discovery that a person with schizophrenia may live in a family who are highly critical, hostile and overinvolved. These families are described as having high expressed emotion. Vaughn and Leff (1976) discovered that when people with schizophrenia were discharged home after a recovery from their symptoms to these families they were more likely to become unwell again even though they were taking medication. Whereas a person with schizophrenia who returned to a family with low expressed emotion was more likely to stay well. These concepts have led to the development of psychosocial interventions and are discussed further in this chapter and also in Chapter 14 of this text.

The stress vulnerability model developed by Zubin and Spring (1977) suggests that people with schizophrenia have genetic and biological vulnerabilities to personal, familial and environmental stressors and that this theory is a way of explaining the onset of schizophrenia and any relapses; therefore, strategies are required to help reduce the impact of stress on them, for example improving coping skills. A result of this is that the person with schizophrenia may feel more equipped to deal with their personal, familial and environmental stressors and less likely to suffer a relapse in their condition.

A study in Edinburgh in 2005 demonstrated:

> People in high-risk categories for schizophrenia go on to develop the disease, show subtle and early warning signs that distinguish them from others in their group. (Johnstone *et al.* 2005).

The study, which began in 1994, tracked 163 young adults identified as 'at risk' of schizophrenia (based on the fact that each subject had two relatives diagnosed with schizophrenia). According to the data, those in this group who developed schizophrenia had more prediagnosed anxiety, social withdrawal and schizotypal thoughts than those who remained well. Such early symptoms were subtle in nature, tending not to be debilitating to daily life.

Given that such problems may develop slowly over several years before they become debilitating, this strongly supports the benefits of early screening, identification and treatment of those who are at genetic and/or environmental risk of developing schizophrenia.

CARE AND TREATMENT

The community treatment team, who can be made available following GP referral, have been recommended to intervene as early as possible. This intervention is supported by the *National Service Framework* (Department of Health 1999), particularly with young people following their first episode of psychosis and confirmation of schizophrenia as a diagnosis. Prompt intervention can reduce morbidity and death rates in youths and in first-episode psychosis has been cited as crucial to an optimistic prognosis of the illness. Prompt and early intervention provides the opportunity to consider real and practical options for successful treatment.

According to Birchwood (1998), there are two main views of schizophrenia. The first is one of early or acute onset psychosis, with frequent bouts or episodes of psychotic features which are followed up by direct treatment, usually medication and some level of recovery, preventive and proactive intervention. The other view is when the intervention is unsuccessful a rehabilitation programme, with psychosocial interventions such as cognitive behavioural therapy (CBT), is helpful. This is an active form of intervention, which deliberately intends to alter thinking and feelings of lack of control to those of empowerment and direct control over one's life. This intervention would run alongside and complement antipsychotic medication. Askey (2002) claims CBT provides hope for people suffering from mental illness. He recommends that mental health practitioners should be prepared to confidently encompass psychosocial interventions into their everyday practice. 'Psychosocial intervention' is a term used to describe interventions that promote engagement with service users. These are directly linked to facilitate family life, for example family therapy, CBT, prompt involvement and response to psychotic episodes. This requires a committed community mental health team with expertise, to be effective, respond quickly to crises and acute episodes.

Peculiar and strange thought patterns are significant signs in the assessment and eventual diagnosis of schizophrenia. These signs and symptoms may be obvious or, alternatively, so subtle that asking and reframing the same questions during the assessment period may eventually unfold the complex world of a person living with schizophrenia. Family and carers are key figures in assisting and unravelling their relative's clinical story. They can participate and provide valuable information prior to the onset of schizophrenia. This can be demonstrated in Scenario Three.

Scenario Three: Assessment of thought patterns

In order for Brian to express his feelings, he began to write in code, which only he understood. It looked like a form of shorthand used by secretaries. When he was asked to decode the writing by the psychiatrist, he began to speak in a strange language when reading it back to her. She asked him to translate the script into English and when he did so the contents were of a sexual nature. He had written in this form for at least seven years and tucked it away under his bed. He had gone through many A4 pads of paper. No one thought it important. The staff observed his behaviour in the confines of the ward but did not think the written scribbles were of any clinical value. They could not see any outward or positive signs of psychosis. Negative symptoms were apparent – lack of drive and motivation and a lack of any insight into his illness. The nurses were looking in the wrong place. Brian's sister asked the psychiatrist to look at her brother's note pads and query their contents.

SOCIAL SKILLS TRAINING AS A THERAPEUTIC INTERVENTION

The negative affects of schizophrenia and psychotic episodes erode the person's confidence and ability to socialise. Their interactive skills become blunted and they become anxious in larger groups and understandably avoid these situations. Social skills training (SST) aims to reduce isolation and loneliness and increase self-confidence and self-esteem. The model developed by Argyle and Kendon (1996) considers social skills training as skills that have to be 'learned and practised', and mental health practitioners are to attempt to identify deficits in service users' social skills. Using role modelling, the practitioners can demonstrate the skills the service user with schizophrenia requires so that they can learn and practice these in everyday life.

Murgatroyd (1985) states that the aims of SST should be:

- to provide a safe environment in which to practise and develop social skills
- to be in a position of a helper/facilitator so that the person with schizophrenia can give feedback; this relationship is vital when providing feedback (the ability to accept constructive criticism comes with confidence building)
- to replicate activities of daily living such as initiating conversation and interacting with others in a safe environment, then repeat these scenarios in real life.

Howard (2002) promotes the use of an 'evening club' within the community which meets one day per week to provide service users with a forum and a bridge between residential and community care. She reports commitment and success from the group, recommending flexibility and creative facilitation as key skills in the process.

ANTIPSYCHOTIC MEDICATION

Chlorpromazine was one of the first antipsychotics and was first used for the treatment of psychoses in 1952. Pharmaceutical companies honed in on the idea of the apparent success of chlorpromazine and promoted their research into brain activity. In particular, a neurotransmitter is responsible for receiving messages that stimulate the production of dopamine, a chemical that, when over produced, is closely linked with schizophrenia.

Gourney (2003) refers to research in an effort to explore the progress into our understanding of treatment methods. He relates it to the acquisition of knowledge, which has increased tremendously over the past two decades; particularly of the major chemical imbalances, or 'chemical chaos', experienced by people with schizophrenia and why the same form of antipsychotic medication may suit one person and be ineffective in another. However, in the main, there appears to be confirmation that people who suffer from schizophrenia respond better to antipsychotics than without them, and particularly to second-generation antipsychotics, or 'atypical neuroleptics'.

Watson (2003) states that the attraction of atypical neuroleptics is their less debilitating side effects, in particular weight gain, dry mouth, facial tics and tremors associated with older forms of antipsychotics. The National Institute for Health and Clinical Excellence (2002) recommends the rights of people with schizophrenia to experience the best possible forms of antipsychotic treatment, psychosocial interventions and medication.

According to Gillam (2002) and Bennett (1999), overall, one antipsychotic appears as effective as the other with varying experience of extra pyramidal side effects (EPSE), e.g. tremors of the hands. The shuffling of feet while trying to maintain a regular normal walking pace is another common symptom (this is usually referred to as 'a shuffling gait'). Raised prolactin, a hormone produced in both males and females, can be overproduced in males, which enlarges breast size in women and occasionally in men and has accompanying weight gain, both of which are very distressing. The person with schizophrenia may experience an excessively dry mouth or excessive saliva production. This can be very distressing as it alters their body image and confidence in everyday activities. It is essential that these symptoms are explained to the person and their families as early detection and reporting assist in a rapid response and review of medication. These symptoms are cited as reasons for non-compliance (non acceptance) with medication. However, the term 'compliance' has been replaced by the term 'concordance' (Norman and Ryrie 2004), which suggests that treatment is an equal partnership based on mutual education and a discussion of the benefits and side effects of medication.

Two examples of antipsychotic medication

Olanzapine (Zyprexa)

This may cause some signs of drowsiness or tiredness, with tendency towards weight gain in the long term. However, there is a low risk associated with EPSE.

Clozapine (Clozaril)

According to Gillam (2002), clozapine should not be used initially as the first drug of choice in first-episode psychosis. Gillam, however, reports success in treatment resistance; when other forms of medication and intervention have had little or no positive effects, he claims it possesses a resistance to sedation/drowsiness. However, it can reduce the production of white blood cells; leading to a low white cell count (agranulocytosis), which ultimately lowers the body's resistance to fight infection, making a person more susceptible to illness. Therefore, early detection is vital and regular blood tests and medication may be reviewed or discontinued. The reported side effects of most antipsychotic medication are (Healy 2005):

- sedation and drowsiness
- lack of motivation
- akinesia – stiffness, lack of movement
- dyskinesia – abnormal movement, usually tremors of the hands or arms that range from fine to severe tremor but may also affect facial muscles
- tardive dyskinesia – late-onset dyskinesia, involuntary abnormal movements of the face and mouth, such as protrusion of the tongue and chewing movements, which may last for several years after stopping taking the medication
- dystonia – a slow movement or extended spasm in a group of muscles
- akathesia – complaints of restlessness accompanied by movements such as, rocking from foot to foot, pacing and being unable to sit still
- orthostatic hypotension – low blood pressure occurs when the person stands up
- dry mouth, constipation
- blurred vision
- urinary retention, urinary incontinence
- skin problems – irritation, rashes
- agranulocytosis – low white cell count
- weight gain
- Neuroleptic Malignant Syndrome – unusually high temperature and flu-like symptoms, with muscle rigidity, requires rapid medical intervention as may be fatal.

These unpleasant side effects impact negatively on people with schizophrenia and can lead to them not taking their medication. Norman and Ryria (2004) use the term 'psychoeducation' to describe improving service users' knowledge about the benefits and side effects of medication. It is an essential part of the role of the practitioner to improve the knowledge not only of the person with schizophrenia but also of their family and therefore allow them to make informed choices about their treatment.

Petit-ZeMan et al. (2002) demonstrate that weight gain is one of the most significant reasons for a service user not taking their medication as they find this weight gain distressing. Facilitation of weight control and overall holistic care is the way forward. Meiklejohn (1999) refers to the physical health in medium secure units as being one of the most neglected areas in clinical practice. This view can be extended to other areas providing health care. Meiklejohn (1999) recommends direct focus on physical health as 'a matter of routine' and that health care practitioners require training in this area in order to be able to offer health promotion advice as a matter of course.

Hannigan and Coffey (2003) report on theories which confirmed that people with schizophrenia were able to predict a relapse in their own mental health. These personal predictions, referred to as 'prodromal signs', alert the service user to the possibility of relapse. They differ from their usual and normal routines; behaviour begins to marginally change from their usual rhythm of life, for example insomnia, increasing levels of anxiety and high or low expressed emotion (extremes of mood) can all be indications of an impending psychotic episode. Recognition of these subtle changes in personal behaviour is the first stage of promoting insight. The person is encouraged to experience a certain level of control over their individual well-being and feel empowered to act on their personal findings. A quick response can minimise the impact of a psychotic episode. Gillam (2002) recommends an 'early warning clinic' for people with schizophrenia to assist one another in identifying and promoting insight and responsibility for themselves.

One mental health promotion strategy could be an advance directive. This is a vehicle that empowers the person with schizophrenia to move quickly to report signs of deterioration. An advance directive is written by the service user and is facilitated by the mental health practitioner. Family members or carers are identified, plus actions the service user wishes to be put into place should they become too ill to make decisions for themselves (Fitzgerald 2001). This advance directive allows the service user, when they are lucid and insightful, to recommend particular personal actions and particular contact persons whom they trust to take care of their home, finances and personal issues. It is not a legally binding document. It can be altered, particularly if the service user becomes so debilitated that they require a formal section of the Mental Health Act 1983 or are detained for treatment.

The advance directive is still a relatively new concept and more needs to be learnt. Rashid (2000) refers to these advance statements as 'living wills', and there are many ethical, legal and administrative issues to explore. These relapse prevention plans (also known as 'relapse signatures') need to be tailored to each person (Kerr 2003). This is a further movement towards partnership and collaboration: the service user and their mental health practitioner can set realistic plans to be put into operation when they are unwell and unable to make decisions about their care and affairs. This is a positive step away from the paternalistic care that many people with schizophrenia have experienced.

CONCLUSION

Schizophrenia is one of the most debilitating forms of enduring mental illness that leaves a person at their most vulnerable and socially isolated. Arguably, schizophrenia and psychosis are the most misunderstood of mental illnesses of the twenty-first century. Surrounded by controversy and provoking debate, fuelled by misrepresentation in the media, this clinical syndrome has a profoundly disparate psychopathology that can severely disrupt the lives of the service users and their families. However, early detection and assessment can ensure the person with schizophrenia and their family receive appropriate care and treatment to promote recovery and develop strategies to maintain health and quality of life.

REFERENCES

Argyle M, Kendon A (1996) In Haddock G, Slade P (eds), *Cognitive Behavioural Interventions with Psychotic Disorders*. London, Routledge.

Askey R (2002) Early onset psychosis: causes and treatment. *Mental Health Practice* 5(10): 16–20.

Barker P (2003) *Psychiatric and Mental Health Nursing: The Craft of Caring*. London, Hodder Arnold.

Bennett J (1999) Antipsychotic Drug Treatment. *Nursing Standard* 13(24): 49–53.

Birchwood M (1998) Early intervention in psychosis: the critical period hypothesis. *International Clinical Pharmacology* 13(suppl 1): 31–40.

Brown GW (1959) Experiences of discharged chronic mental hospital patients in various types of living group. *Millbank Memorial Fund Quarterly* 37: 105–131.

Department of Health (1999) *National Service Frameworks for Mental Health*. London, The Stationery Office.

Donnellan C (2000) *Dealing with Mental Illness*. Cambridge, Independence.

Eby L, Brown NJ (2005) *Mental Health Nursing Care*. Upper Saddle River, NJ, Pearson/Prentice Hall.

Fitzgerald PB (2001) The role of early warning symptoms in the detection and prevention of schizophrenia. *Australian and New Zealand Journal of Psychiatry* 35(6): 758–764.

Fontaine K (2003) *Mental Health Nursing* (5th edn.). Upper Saddle River, NJ, Prentice Hall.

Gelder M, Mayou R, Cowen P (2001) *Shorter Oxford Textbook of Psychiatry*. Oxford, Oxford University Press.

Gillam T (2002) 'Treating' how psychosocial interventions can complement medication. *Mental Health Practice* 6(4): 28–32.

Gourney K (2003) Drug treatments for schizophrenia: why they offer the only hope for patients. *Mental Health Practice* 6(6): 16–17.

Hannigan B, Coffey M (2003) *The Handbook of Community Mental Health Nursing*. London, Routledge.

Healy D (2005) *Psychiatric Drugs Explained* (4th edn.). London, Churchill Livingstone.

Howard V (2002) One of the gang. *Mental Health Practice* 6(3): 6–11.

Johnstone EC, Ebmeier KP, Miller P, Owens DGC, Lawrie SM (2005) Predicting schizophrenia: findings from the Edinburgh High-Risk Study. *British Journal of Psychiatry* 186(Jan): 18–25.

Jones A (2004) Matter over mind: physical wellbeing for people with severe mental illness. *Mental Health Practice* 7(10): 36–38.

Kerr S (2003) *Schizophrenia: Aspects of Care*. London, Whurr.

Kneisl CR, Wilson HS, Trigoboff E (2004) *Contemporary Psychiatric-Mental Health Nursing*. Upper Saddle River, NJ, Pearson/Prentice Hall.

Meiklejohn C (1999) Physical health in medium secure services. *Mental Health Practice* 17(17): 33–37.

Murgatroyd S (1985) *Counselling and Helping*. London, Routledge.

National Institute for Health and Clinical Excellence (2002) *Schizophrenia: Core Interventions in the Treatment and Management of Schizophrenia in Primary and Secondary Care*. London, National Institute for Health and Clinical Excellence.

Norman I, Ryrie I (2004) *The Art and Science of Mental Health Nursing: A Textbook of Principles and Practice*. Maidenhead, Open University Press.

Petit-ZeMan S, Sandamas G, Hogman G (2002) Doesn't It Make You Sick? Side Effects of Medicine and Physical Health Concerns of People with Severe Mental Illness, http://www.rethink.org/applications/site_search/search.rm?term=Petite-Zeman& searchreferer_id=6&submit.x=12&submit.y=16, accessed 18 July 2006.

Rashid C (2000) Philosophical implications of the use of advance statements (living wills). *Nursing Standard* **14**(25): 37–40.

Semple D, Smyth R, Burns J, Darjee R, McIntosh A (2005) *Oxford Textbook of Psychiatry*. Oxford, Oxford University Press.

Social Exclusion Unit (2004) *Mental Health and Social Exclusion*. London, Office of the Deputy Prime Minister.

Sims A (1995) *Symptoms in the Mind* (2nd edn.). London, WD Saunders.

Stuart WG, Laraia MT (2005) *Principles and Practice of Psychiatric Nursing* (8th edn.). St Louis, Elsevier Mosby.

Thomson T, Mathias P (2003) *Lyttle's Mental Health and Disorder*. London, Balliere Tindall.

Vaughn CE, Leff JP (1976) The influence of family life and social factors on the course of psychiatric illness: a comparison of schizophrenic and depressed neurotic patients. *British Journal of Psychiatry* **129**(Aug): 125–137.

Watson D (2003) The psychopharmacological treatment of schizophrenia. *Mental Health Practice* **6**(6): 32–51.

World Health Organization (1992) *The ICD-10 Classification of Mental and Behavioural Disorders*. Geneva, World Health Organization.

Zubin J, Spring B (1977) Vulnerability: a new view of schizophrenia. *Journal of Abnormal Psychology* **86**(2): 103–126.

12 Personality Disorder

B. THOMSON

INTRODUCTION

The aims of this chapter are to describe personality disorder, discuss the diagnostic criteria and the problems associated with the current definitions and to consider various models of personality disorder. Although this chapter will outline currently used diagnostic criteria, the focus will be to describe personality disorder using both user perspectives and the experience of the author to encourage the reader to develop a deeper understanding of the condition.

DEFINING PERSONALITY DISORDER

Definitions of personality disorder are complex. Mental health professionals have a variety of views and attitudes towards personality disorder, and there are many myths and misunderstandings surrounding the issue. However, people with personality disorder make up a large portion of the population who use mental health services. It is estimated that between 36% and 67% of those using mental health services have personality disorder (National Institute for Mental Health in England 2003).

Many service users with personality disorder are dissatisfied with the services available and much has been written about the negative impact of the label 'personality disorder'. Castillo (2003) refers to personality disorder as 'a dangerous diagnosis' and goes on to report the negative impact of such a diagnosis together with the negative attitude of some mental health professionals towards those with the diagnosis.

It is generally accepted among mental health professionals that the therapeutic relationship is fundamental to successfully working with people who have mental health problems. Two crucial aspects of the therapeutic relationship developed in the 1930s by Karl Rogers are 'a non-judgemental attitude' and 'unconditional positive regard', which refers to a positive and respectful attitude towards the patient being an essential element of any successful therapeutic relationship.

Caring for Adults with Mental Health Problems   Edited by I. Peate and S. Chelvanayagam
© 2006 John Wiley & Sons, Ltd

These principles become simultaneously more difficult to sustain yet even more crucial when dealing with some of the challenging behaviour commonly seen in people with a personality disorder. Many of the negative attitudes seen among mental health professionals are the result of a lack of understanding of personality disorder. The predominance of the medical model and the long-held view that these disorders are untreatable further add to the stigma and negative impact of these disorders.

It is hoped that developing a deeper understanding of these behaviours will assist both those working with these disorders and those suffering from the disorders to be more understanding and to maintain a more positive attitude. Having an understanding of and correctly interpreting of behaviours seen in personality disorder are essential for a successful treatment plan. Many of the most successful treatments for personality disorder contain a large element of education, self-awareness and social skills training (Linehan 1993).

HOW PERSONALITY DISORDER IS CLASSIFIED

The *International Classification of Mental and Behavioural Disorders* (*ICD-10*) defines a personality disorder as:

> A severe disturbance in the Carachterological condition and behavioural tendencies of the individual usually involving several areas of the personality and nearly always associated with considerable personal and social disruption. (World Health Organization 1992).

The fourth edition of the *Diagnostic and Statistical Manual of Mental Disorders* (*DSM-IV*) defines personality disorders as:

> An enduring pattern of inner experience and behaviour that deviates markedly from the expectations of the individual's culture, is pervasive and inflexible, has an onset in adolescence or early adulthood, is stable over time, and leads to distress or impairment. (American Psychiatric Association 1994).

It could be suggested that these definitions are imprecise and open to interpretation. This has led to difficulties with diagnosis. These diagnostic criteria are even less helpful as a description of the problem, both for health care professionals and for those diagnosed with these disorders.

MacFarlane (2004) suggests that researchers have found a high incidence of overlap between the different categories. There has been much discussion of problems using these diagnostic criteria, for example when a person with a personality disorder does not meet the full criteria for any one diagnosis but nonetheless has a significant impairment and symptoms spread across several different categories.

Another fundamental problem with these criteria is that many of the traits discussed can be seen in most people at times, for example manipulation, emotional coldness and suspiciousness can all be seen in the general population. Therefore, it becomes necessary to ask at what point this should be seen as a symptom of personality disorder and not just a personality trait within the bounds of normality. Other criticisms include a lack of consistent theoretical basis for understanding the aetiology of these conditions and a lack of significance in terms of treatment planning or clinical interventions. Certainly, the long-held belief that these conditions were part of a person's personality and therefore fixed and untreatable has been disproved (National Institute for Mental Health in England 2003).

There are nine categories of *ICD-10* personality disorder and ten categories of *DSM-IV* personality disorder. These classification schemes should be treated with caution as patients with personality disorder can often be fitted into several different categories and many of the behaviours described can be observed in many healthy people.

The *DSM-IV* attempts to simplify things by grouping the subcategories into three broad clusters:

1. Cluster A (odd or eccentric types): paranoid, schizoid and schizotypal. **Traits**: suspicious, bears grudges, tenacious, litigious, paranoid, emotionally cold, solitary, indifferent to others' views, odd beliefs, ideas of reference, socially withdrawn.
2. Cluster B (dramatic, emotional or erratic types): histrionic, narcissistic, antisocial and borderline. **Traits**: unstable relationships, low self-esteem, impulsivity, repetitive suicidal or self-harm behaviour, mood fluctuations, deceitfulness, lying, reckless, antisocial behaviour, overdramatic, attention-seeking, seductive, shallow, self-important, need for admiration, grandiose.
3. Cluster C (anxious and fearful types): obsessive-compulsive, avoidant and dependent. **Traits**: submissive, clinging, fear of separation, excessive need for others to take responsibility for them, hypersensitive, inadequate, orderly, need for rules and order, pedantic, rigid, stubborn, cautious, obsessive.

It is a matter of severity of the dysfunctional responses and behaviours coupled to the fact that these dysfunctional patterns have an enduring quality. It is important to note, however, that current research demonstrates that with the appropriate treatment people can recover from personality disorder – although, despite the mounting body of evidence, this remains a controversial issue.

ALTERNATIVE MODELS

DIMENSIONAL MODEL

Other health care professionals have developed models of personality based on various psychological theories. One dimensional model described by Costa and

McCrae (1992) sees personality disorders as part of a continuum of normal personality traits. They describe a 'five factor model'. The five core personality traits identified in this model are:

- neuroticism
- extraversion
- openness
- agreeableness
- conscientiousness.

In this model, personality disorder symptoms are seen as being at the extremes of these traits.

PROTOTYPICAL CLASSIFICATION SYSTEM

Millon and Davis (1995) developed a model known as the prototypical classification system. This combines the strengths of the *DSM* classifications with the dimensional system. The authors recommend the clinician asks both 'how' and 'how much' questions regarding symptoms. Using this method, patients falling below the *DSM* classification are still included in the model.

STRUCTURAL DYNAMIC CLASSIFICATION

Psychoanalysts describe the structural dynamic classification model. This model is based on psychoanalytic character types and arranges personality on a structural continuum: normal, neurotic borderline and psychotic (McWilliams 1994).

RELATIONAL CLASSIFICATION

Magnavita (2000) attempts to fit personality traits into a relational classification model. This model sees personality disorders as dysfunctional personality systems that exist between interpersonal relationships. In other words, the symptoms develop within dysfunctional relationships and are then carried forward into subsequent relationships.

COGNITIVE MODEL

Beck and Freeman (1990) propose a cognitive behavioural understanding of personality disorder. This model conceptualises personality disorder as a set of core beliefs and dysfunctional assumptions that are consolidated into a personal schema, that is a mind set of core beliefs which influence our perceptions and the way we make sense of the world.

These faulty schemata are maintained by cognitive distortions leading to problematic behaviours. The main advantage of this model is that it provides a framework which can be used to develop treatments. Cognitive behavioural therapy techniques have been identified as among the most effective interventions for the treatment of personality disorder.

A SERVICE USER MODEL

Among service users with personality disorder, there is a view that personality disorder may be a type of long-term post-traumatic stress disorder. This way of understanding personality disorder can be useful as it is a popular viewpoint among service users. It could be argued that trauma or severe distress can interfere with the normal development of various personality traits and skills; this leaves open the possibility of recovery. Once the trauma has been dealt with, the person can learn and experience personal growth and can develop skills and personality.

COMMON PRESENTATIONS IN PERSONALITY DISORDER

The following descriptions are based on observations and discussions with people suffering from personality disorder and rely heavily on the courage and honesty of many clients both during therapy and in service user forums.

Personality disorder has its roots in childhood and adolescence, when the personality is developing (Bloom 1997). Commonly, those with personality disorder have experienced prolonged abuse or emotional disturbance, which appear to interfere with the development of a healthy personality complete with the coping mechanisms and social skills necessary for healthy relationships and interactions in society.

It is important to note that, although sexual, physical and emotional abuse and neglect are common, sometimes a fragile child perceives rejection and abuse in the absence of actual abuse, see the scenario below.

Scenario One

Clair was brought up in a home with a father who was withdrawn and emotionally unavailable, as he was suffering from depression. Clair believed her father avoided her because she was somehow flawed and unlovable. In fact, her father feared passing on his depression and avoided her in order to protect her. Her mother worked long hours to provide for the family, leaving her in the care of her grandmother. After her grandmother's death, when Clair was 13, Clair felt abandoned and alone. Once this belief of being unlovable was fixed in her mind, it began to affect the way she perceived the world and coloured all her interactions with people. Her self-esteem sank to a level that made it impossible for her to have normal healthy relationships with anyone, and over a period of years she deteriorated to a level where she could barely function. She hated herself and felt continuously suicidal. Clair also felt intense anger at her parents and had made life very difficult for them. Despite this, Clair's parents continued to love and support her in many ways. Clair, however, could not see this and continued to believe she was unloved.

FEATURES OF PERSONALITY DISORDER

One defining characteristic of personality disorder is the intense discomfort with one's own emotional responses to certain trigger situations. This inevitably leads to dysfunctional behaviours. From the frantic efforts of the borderline to avoid the intense emotional distress to the cold denial and dissociation of the antisocial, the common factor is an overwhelmingly fearful, often phobic, response to their own emotions: this is described as 'frozen terror' (Johnson 2000).

For the health care professional, it is always a good idea to keep a note of trigger situations. These will usually have some common themes that, once identified, act as arrows pointing to specific vulnerabilities. Psychotherapeutic input can then be targeted towards the relevant issues.

Another common factor is an incredibly low self-esteem (in some people this is hidden under a façade of superiority). This is often the result of years of invalidating experiences, leading many people with personality disorder to believe that they are bad, worthless, evil or unacceptable in some way.

Those who suffer from this debilitating belief will often find it excruciatingly uncomfortable to receive compliments, since anything positive said about them conflicts with their established self-image. This discomfort often leads to dysfunctional behaviours, and they regard the person giving the compliment with suspicion. For example, if you 'know' what someone is saying is obviously untrue, it is only logical to be suspicious as to why they are saying it.

People with personality disorder can alternate between avoiding others (because they know they will be rejected) or desperately clinging onto a relationship in an inappropriate manner in an attempt to avoid the overwhelming emotional hurt of facing rejection yet again, which will confirm all their worst fears about themselves.

Most people have felt the pain of rejection at some time in their lives. For people with personality disorder, the feelings evoked by these situations (hurt, anguish, self-loathing and despair) can be overwhelming. The fear of what they might do in these circumstances is often terrifying, and with good cause. People with personality disorder are more likely to commit suicide than any other group (MacFarlane 2004).

Moskovitz (1996) describes borderline personality disorder as 'emotional haemophilia'. He suggests that if you prick a person with personality disorder emotionally they may bleed to death emotionally. It is important to recognise that once people have experienced this pain a few times they become extremely sensitive to rejection and it becomes so important to avoid it happening again that they become hypervigilant and develop strategies to predict and avoid any situation that might trigger these emotions.

Small things can trigger a huge response. Anything from not talking to them, or failing to phone as arranged, to telling them you are too busy to see them can be perceived by them as proof that they are worthless and unlovable and can trigger a response that is literally life-threatening.

This can be misunderstood by health care professionals, who perceive this as 'acting out' or manipulative behaviour. One common response to these behaviours is to attempt to discourage them by ignoring them. This crude behavioural response is never effective; if a client is seeking attention, it may be because they need more attention. To deprive them of attention therefore will most likely lead to more desperate attention-seeking behaviours and may damage the therapeutic relationship.

The effect of withholding attention from the client at a time when they feel a desperate need for attention may well be to confirm their belief that no one cares and thus reinforce their underlying schema that they are worthless and not deserving of any understanding or care.

A far better strategy in these situations is to provide the necessary attention at the time, then at a time when the client is calm and secure use the incident to discuss with the client what happened and then to teach them more appropriate ways of meeting their needs when they find themselves in this type of situation. These socioeducational interventions can be among the most helpful interventions for treating personality disorder.

People with this personality disorder are extremely sensitive. They are expert at picking up the tiniest clue such as body language or tone of voice posture or facial expression. Often, these people have an exceptional ability to pick up on others' feelings and will often be the first to notice if a fellow service user is feeling low, angry, suicidal or upset. Sadly, although so often accurate and understanding towards other people's emotional turmoil, when it comes to their own they may be blinded by their negative beliefs about themselves and so closed to any interpretation other than the worst.

Common responses to these sensitivities vary from person to person and from time to time; however, it may be useful to discuss a few behaviours that are often seen and repeated many times among this client group.

SOME FEATURES ASSOCIATED WITH PERSONALITY DISORDER

There is a group of behaviours that, although seen in normal healthy interactions, are taken to extremes or carried out in an inappropriate manner by those with personality disorder. These are:

- always being nice to everyone
- ignoring one's own needs and putting everyone else first
- never letting people know if they upset you
- becoming overinvolved in other people's problems
- developing close relationships in a rushed or superficial way.

There is also another group of behaviours that range from frantic attempts to control or avoid situations to paradoxical behaviours designed to take the sting out of a situation by making it happen before it occurs.

Frantic or hysterical reactions to real or imagined rejection or abandonment   For example, one client swallowed her husband's car keys when she became convinced he would leave her after they had an argument. Another clung to his legs as he attempted to leave screaming that she would kill herself if he left.

Apologising inappropriately and taking the blame for others to avoid confrontation or its consequences   A female client who had been abused and undermined for many years by her husband not only stayed with him but covered up for him and made excuses for his behaviour always saying it was her fault or that she had made him hit her.

Shooting yourself in the foot   A male client panicked so much if he enjoyed anything that he would sabotage anything he enjoyed because he was convinced that he would lose it in the end.

Testing out   This is where clients provoke rejection in order to prove to themselves that they are right in their suspicions that they are going to be rejected. They often push and push at friends, family or professionals in order to prove that their fears of rejection are correct.

Anyone who they fear may reject or abandon them will be subjected to a series of tests where they will provoke the very rejection they fear. Unfortunately, these fears and beliefs appear to be so ingrained that no amount of acceptance, tolerance or evidence is sufficient to offer reassurance, and this 'testing out process' often continues unabated.

A more problematic form of this that is seen in antisocial personality disorder is when the client purposely behaves in an antisocial or objectionable manner. This appears to be an attempt to gain control over the rejection, for example if you intentionally make people dislike or reject you, it can take the sting out of the rejection as you do not have to face the heartache of being disliked or rejected when you are attempting to be accepted or liked.

Testing fate   In extreme circumstances, clients will sometimes indulge in dangerous death-defying behaviour. One client, when very distressed, would play chicken on the road with trucks. Her reasoning was 'Well, if I die, I don't care; if I don't die, that means I'm supposed to carry on.' Often the highly dangerous nature of these behaviours creates a state of high arousal and excitement that distracts the person from the distress of the trigger situation. These dysfunctional responses to emotional distress are the key to understanding personality disorder. The sheer terror and extreme distress that can suddenly overwhelm a person with personality disorder is the primary cause of most of the problems experienced by this group.

These highly emotional states can be triggered very suddenly and at these times the person may feel totally out of control. They develop patterns of behaviour to cope with these emotional overload situations. Self-harm, suicide, violence – anything is better than having to face the emotion.

Often people with personality disorder feel that they have no choice in these situations. They are out of control and need someone else to keep them safe and help them regain control. In some extreme cases, the person dissociates themselves from the situation so completely that they are unaware of what they are doing. Sometimes, after the event they will have no memory of what has happened.

Black-and-white thinking   The world is a really inconsistent place. People have good and bad moods; they may do and say nice things one moment and bad things on another occasion. For people with personality disorder, this is really confusing because these inconsistencies do not fit with the way they perceive the world. This leads to a process known as 'splitting', where everything gets divided into extremes and only one extreme is perceived at any one time.

Making judgements becomes very difficult as the judgement will not be made in a balanced way but will depend on which extreme is being perceived at that moment. This in turn may mean that the judgement will change when the perception changes. People with this problem are often aware that they have difficulty making judgements and learn not to trust their own judgement as a result.

Black-and-white thinking does not just apply to people; it can apply to anything. For example, Angela, a client with borderline personality disorder, could not understand how she could believe anything good about herself without becoming horrendously arrogant; as she really hated the idea of being arrogant, she refused to believe anything good about herself.

This leads to a bizarre perception of the world. Everything is black or white and what was once black can become white, but by the time it does the client cannot remember how it appeared when it was black and it may then switch back again. This inconsistent perception leads to feelings of insecurity and confusion. It is very difficult to live in a world that changes all the time, and making decisions becomes impossible.

Splitting   This term is used to describe the process where people with personality disorder split off different parts of their own personality. In extreme cases, this splitting is so extreme that the person may have no memory of what they have been doing in one mode when they are in another. In the US, this is sometimes seen as 'multiple personality disorder'. However, these 'personalities' are incomplete fragments of personality rather than complete and distinct personalities in themselves. In the UK, the same presentation is seen as dissociation in a fragmented personality. Either way, treatment is aimed at consolidating the various aspects into one complete person. The scenario below provides an example.

Scenario Two

Sue, a client with bipolar disorder, was feeling very unsafe and desperately trying to get admitted to the acute mental health admission ward. She was repeatedly phoning various health care professionals saying that she was feeling suicidal and would kill herself if they did not admit her.

However, when she was offered a job interview in the middle of all this, she split into a different mode of her personality and not only attended the interview but was able to act and behave in a calm, professional manner and was offered a high-powered job. After the interview, she immediately switched back to her previous needy mode and continued her attempts to be admitted to the acute mental health admission ward.

This apparent contradiction was interpreted by some staff as proof that she was being manipulative and that her need was not genuine. In reality, there was no contradiction, as Sue had automatically switched to a different mode, one which was necessary to attend the interview that was important to her. This splitting is not under the conscious control of the client and can be as confusing to the person suffering from this symptom as it is to their family and carers.

Lack of 'core identity' People with personality disorder often have difficulty understanding who they really are. Often they describe feeling like they are nothing or nobody. In a healthy personality, people develop traits and choose values in response to their experiences. They choose what aspects of society and culture are important to them. Over time, these choices become integrated into their personality, part of who they are.

A client with personality disorder is often hyper-aware of this process and interprets it as being somehow fake or unreal. This leads to excessive introspection and self-criticism, which significantly contributes to the dysfunctionality of the client with personality disorder.

Clients with these symptoms are often social chameleons, adapting who they are, their likes, dislikes and preferences to fit in with those around them. This is often an attempt to fit in and be accepted, or to disguise their sense of being 'no one'. However, this leads to further feelings of being a fraud. It is hard to be yourself if you have no idea of who 'you' are.

This process of inconsistent personal identity also makes it easy to dismiss any positive feedback from other people. If they are not seeing the real you, their positive comments are not genuinely about you but only comments regarding the person you are pretending to be. Interestingly, this does not seem to hold true for negative comments. These tend to be interpreted as insightful perceptions seeing through the attempts to appear acceptable.

One major difficulty this causes is that clients with personality disorder will often 'become' the client that health care professionals expect, that is anorexic, addict, psychotic, depressed. Often it is only after several failed treatment programmes that the health care professionals begin to question their original diagnosis.

This can lead to further difficulties when the client loses confidence in the health care professional's ability to understand or help them. Some will see this as evidence that health care professionals are easily fooled; for others it only serves to strengthen their belief that they are beyond help and utterly hopeless.

Self-harm This symptom is so common among those with personality disorder that to some health care professionals it has become almost diagnostic of personality disorder. This is a dangerous simplification for, although it is true that many people who have personality disorder do self-harm, there are many people who self-harm that do not have a personality disorder, and vice versa.

When discussing self-harm, it is important to recognise that this does not include suicidal behaviour. These two are often discussed as if they are varying levels of the same thing. This is a not the case. Self-harm has several functions not related to suicide. It is important to differentiate the two in order to maintain an accurate assessment of risk and formulate appropriate responses and treatment plans.

For those who suffer from personality disorder, self-harm is a coping mechanism. For some, far from being life-threatening, self-harm is an attempt to gain sufficient control to avoid committing suicide (Scenario three).

Scenario Three

Catherine was a woman with a long history of sexual abuse in her childhood. When these memories were triggered, she would become very distressed and obsessed with self-loathing and self-hatred. If left unabated, this self-hatred would become so distressing that she would see no other way to end the distress other than suicide. These feelings would become so unbearable that Catherine knew from her experience she would eventually attempt to kill herself to end the pain. The only reliable method she had found to dissipate her obsessive rumination and self-loathing was to burn her arms with cigarettes.

As can be seen from the above scenario, for Catherine self-harm was an attempt to stop her from committing suicide. This type of self-harm is a life-saving coping strategy. It is not surprising therefore that clients are loath to give it up, especially before they have been taught how to develop alternative strategies to use in these situations.

People self-harm for a many reasons; however, most of them are attempts at expressing or enduring strong emotions. It is important when working with people with personality disorder to work with them towards a clear understanding of their personal beliefs and reasons underpinning the self-harm. Only in this way can you begin to develop alternative strategies that once in place enable the client to reduce the frequency and intensity of their self-harm.

For most, self-harm will decrease or stop of its own accord once alternatives are in place, certainly attempts to stop self-harm before alternatives are in place are doomed to failure as patients will be reluctant to give up their coping strategy until they have an alternative. Initial interventions should therefore be aimed at limiting the dangerousness of the self-harm and encouraging the client to manage their behaviour rather than stop it.

Some clinicians have speculated that self-harm creates an adrenaline rush causing a sort of high. Others believe that the pain leads to a release of endorphins in the brain, which helps to restore a feeling of calm and well-being. Regardless of the theoretical approach taken, it becomes clear that self-harm is a very complex and individual process: some clients describe it as self-punishment; others as a release of pressures or to see blood flow or understand their self-harm in terms of 'letting the evil out'.

To work successfully with self-harm, it is necessary to work collaboratively with the client to understand their underlying schema. Only then can the health care professional hope to develop interventions that will be successful in treating this distressing condition.

Mood instability   This is a chronic problem for people with personality disorder. Relatively small things can have huge consequences. This causes further problems for the person who cannot explain their emotions in terms of an understandable response to circumstances. This leads to one of the most difficult presentations seen in personality disorder: 'exaggerations and untruths'. People with personality disorder often talk in parables. They will tell you a story that explains or accounts for the way they feel. The following scenario illustrates this.

Scenario Four

Alison was a woman who had suffered multiple sexual abuses throughout her life. She was so damaged by these that she viewed any sexual advances or behaviours as assaults and was totally unable to understand healthy sexual desire or activity. While travelling on a bus one day, she noticed a male passenger looking at her. Immediately, she interpreted this as a danger signal. She felt that she was being assaulted and became extremely distressed.

She went to the community centre for support. However, she knew that she could not explain her extreme emotional distress in terms of the truth (i.e. a man on the bus looked at me). Therefore, in order to make sense of her distress and get the support she needed, Alison told the staff that a man sexually assaulted her on the bus.

Although not literally true, the emotions behind this event were true.

Since it is often impossible to determine the underlying truth in these situations, the health care professional is in a position where it becomes impossible to be sure about what actions are appropriate Therefore, in these situations it is important to focus on the needs of the person rather than respond to the literal presentation.

In Alison's case, for example, if the staff respond to the emotional need they will be able to give Alison the support she needs and dissipate the situation; if however, they respond to the situation they may have involved the police or bus company leading to more stress and problems for Alison, who would be left having to elaborate on her story – and possibly even being caught out lying, leading to more distress and self-loathing. This process often damages the therapeutic relationship and exacerbates the whole situation.

While dealing with these situations, especially in the early stages of treatment, it is better not to 'add insight to injury' and instead simply address the emotion behind the story and look to meet the 'expressed need'. Later on in the treatment process, the client can be supported to understand this process and moderate their behaviours accordingly. Until this level of understanding and social skill is achieved, it is best to offer support to your client without either challenging or acting on the story itself.

Anger   This can be a huge problem for those with personality disorder. Both over-expression or under-expression can be the problem for this group of clients. Both can occur in the same person at the same time. Those with personality disorder often have a heightened sense of injustice and will often be the first to respond if they see someone else being unfairly treated or abused.

However, when the injustice or abuse is aimed at them, they rarely manage to be as vocal or stand up for themselves in the way they do for others. This is often because their self-esteem is so low and self-image is either that they deserve the abuse or that they are powerless to prevent it. This acceptance of abuse further undermines their self-image and self-confidence and they often misinterpret it as 'What I deserve or all I can expect'.

Some clients are so fearful of what they might do if they ever gave vent to their feelings of anger that they have learnt to repress these feelings completely. This fear of losing control is a major inhibitor when it comes to working with clients to help them recognise their emotions and deal with them appropriately, as clients who exhibit this symptom have great difficulty when it comes to being aware of their feelings.

Other commonalities found in people suffering from personality disorder but not included in any of the diagnostic models are listed below.

The ability to appear normal   This can be very difficult for everyone concerned, as people with personality disorder can act normally for large parts of the time; the illness often goes unrecognised for a long time. Even the person themselves can fail to recognise that they have a mental disorder. Often, they just see themselves as weak, useless, unlovable or stupid. Sometimes, it comes as a great relief to be diagnosed and told that there is actually something wrong and that they can be helped.

Memory problems   These are extremely common among this group. This can be due to dissociation, but more often than not it is just that there is too much going on in their minds at any one time. This can be anything from self-chastisement and hypervigilance to full-blown psychotic hallucinations. This preoccupation makes it difficult to concentrate or focus normally.

Insecurity or fear of change   This is another common problem for those with personality disorder. Often, the person can be affected by staff changes or disruptions to routines. Fairly minor changes can have a huge effect on their confidence or ability to function.

Sleep disturbance or nightmares   These are common problems often experienced by people with personality disorder. The night-time can be a very difficult period when left with no distractions: alone with their thoughts, the patient may often find themselves desperate for morning. Yet when it arrives they are so tired as a result of their nocturnal ruminations that they are desperate for night to come. This relentless pattern can, when severe, lead to a total breakdown.

Dependence   This can often be heard as an excuse used to avoid offering help to people with personality disorder. Some health care professionals may fear offering services in case it promotes dependence. While dependence can be a genuine problem at times, it is a necessary part of the healing process. Dependence can best be viewed as a stage between total chaos and independence. Without going through a period of dependency, the person with personality disorder may never become truly independent. The role of the mental health professional is to be dependable and consistent in their support and acceptance of their clients.

People with these disorders often suffer from a variety of symptoms common in other mental illnesses. They can have another illness alongside their personality disorder. However, more commonly, they may experience several symptoms from a variety of illnesses. This often leads to a number of misdiagnoses before they are eventually diagnosed with personality disorder.

MEDICATION

The symptoms described above can respond well to symptomatic treatment with the relevant drugs. For example, someone who experiences psychotic symptoms such as hallucinations may respond well to a short course of antipsychotic medication; however, prophylactic use of these drugs is often unsuccessful and so patients are usually given a small amount to use when these symptoms occur. This is often a more acceptable use of medication for people with personality disorders who dislike being on medication or fear its side effects. It also has the additional benefit of enabling the client to take some control over their treatment, which helps promote self-reliance.

Mood swings in personality disorder must be distinguished from bipolar disorder. If a mood chart is kept, there may be a pattern to the mood swings in bipolar disorder, whereas in personality disorder mood swings are often triggered by events and so appear more random; often these can be seen to result from dissociation or splitting.

Semisodium valporate (Depakote) can be very helpful in dealing with the very intense emotional distress seen in these clients. Many clients find this drug lowers the intensity of their emotions and gives them back the emotional control they so fear losing. Other medications, such as antidepressants, can be helpful but are not an answer in themselves. Rather, these can most helpfully be viewed as a crutch to support the client while therapeutic interventions are used to help them develop healthy psychological mechanisms and social skills. When using medication, it must always be remembered that these clients have a higher risk of suicide than any other group. Care must be taken to ensure medication is not misused or saved up for use in an unhealthy manner.

Addictive behaviour is another common problem for this group. The excessive use of alcohol and recreational drugs is commonly used by this group as a desperate measure to escape from their distress. Although reducing these behaviours may be an appropriate short-term goal during therapy, these people with personality disorders are significantly different from other drug users. Often, if you address the root cause or motivating factors, drug or alcohol use is no longer needed and ceases to be a problem.

CONCLUSION

Personality disorder can be a frustrating, disabling and confusing condition for the client and for those working with them. Progress can be turbulent and erratic with many pitfalls and problems to be overcome along the way. However, with genuine collaboration, honesty and mutual respect, people with personality disorder can learn to live full and productive lives. Once set free from their emotional turmoil and destructive behaviours, people with personality disorders can learn that they are not the misfits they may have thought they were and can go on to make peace with themselves and the world around them.

In many cases, people with a personality disorder have survived the worst this world can throw at them. They may have been damaged or seriously affected by their life experiences, but they are survivors. They deserve respect as well as a professional approach to their care. With patience, practice and perseverance, health care professionals can have the privilege of getting close enough to help the person with personality disorder achieve this.

REFERENCES

American Psychiatric Association (1994) *Diagnostic and Statistical Manual of Mental Disorders*. Washington, American Psychiatric Association.

Beck AT, Freeman A (1990) *Cognitive Therapy of Personality Disorders*. New York, Guilford Press.

Bloom S (1997) *Creating Sanctuary: Towards the Evolution of Sane Societies*. New York, Routledge.

Castillo H (2003) A dangerous diagnosis. *Mental Health Today* February: 27–30.

Costa PT, McCrae RR (1992) The five factor model of personality disorder and its relevance to personality disorders. *Journal of Personality Disorders* **6**: 343–359.

Johnson B (2002) *Emotional Health*. York, James Nayler Foundation.

Linehan MM (1993) *The Skills Training Manual for Treating Borderline Personality Disorder*. New York, Guilford Press.

MacFarlane M (2004) *Family Treatment of Personality Disorder*. New York, Haworth Clinical Practice Press.

Magnavita JJ (2000) *Relational Therapy for Personality Disorders*. New York, John Wiley & Sons.

McWilliams (1994) *Psychoanalytic Diagnosis: Understanding Personality Structure in Clinical Practice*. New York, Guilford Press.

Millon T, Davies RD (1995) Conceptions of personality disorders: the DSM and future directions. In Livesley WJ (ed), *The DSM IV Personality Disorders*. New York, Guilford Press, pp. 3–27.

Moskovitz R (1996) *Lost in the Mirror: An Inside Look at Borderline Personality Disorder*. Dallas, TX, Taylor Trade.

National Institute for Mental Health in England (2003) *Report on Personality Disorder: No Longer a Diagnosis of Exclusion*. London, The Stationery Office.

World Health Organization (1992) *International Classification of Mental and Behavioural Disorders*. Geneva, World Health Organization.

13 Dementias

S. HAHN

INTRODUCTION

This chapter aims to provide information on different types of dementia and how people with dementia and their families can be supported effectively. By understanding the way dementia may affect someone's life, staff are more able to provide care that will be empowering and appropriate to the needs of the individual and their family.

The Alzheimer's Society defines dementia as:

> The loss of intellectual functions (such as thinking, remembering, and reasoning) of sufficient severity to interfere with a person's daily functioning. (Alzheimer's Society 2006a).

Dementia is not a disease itself but a group of symptoms that may include changes in personality, mood and behaviour. Dementia is irreversible when caused by disease or injury but may be reversible when caused by drugs, alcohol, hormone or vitamin imbalances or depression.

The term 'dementia' tends to raise a variety of thoughts and feelings for people. Some may be based on experience, either personal or professional, and some on common myths and misunderstandings. The important thing is to understand the different ways in which dementia can develop and the impact it may have upon the individual and those close to them (Cheston & Bender 1999).

For too long, people with dementia were seen as not having the ability to make decisions about their future and so have often been excluded from the diagnosis and treatment, or care, plans. The advent of drugs such as Aricept and Exelon has encouraged earlier assessment and given greater hope to people with dementia of the possibility that the progress of dementia may be slowed (Bender 1999). If people with dementia are to receive high-quality care, it is important to develop an understanding of the ways in which information, respect and communication affect the care given to and received by people with dementia and their families.

Dementia affects 750,000 people in the UK, and it is estimated that this will increase to 870,000 by 2010, and to 1.8 million by 2050 (Alzheimer's Society

Caring for Adults with Mental Health Problems   Edited by I. Peate and S. Chelvanayagam
© 2006 John Wiley & Sons, Ltd

2006b). The rise in the number of people with dementia is not confined to the UK; it is happening worldwide. There are 18 million people across the world with dementia, and it is estimated that by 2025 this number will increase to 34 million (Alzheimer's Society 2006b). Seventy-one per cent will be in countries of poor or middle income, such as some of those in Africa and Asia. This increase is directly associated with the ageing population, as the incidence of dementia increases with age. In people over the age of 65 years, one in 20 is affected by dementia, increasing to 1 person in five over the age of 80 years (Alzheimer's Society 2006b).

'Dementia' is a general term used to describe various brain disorders that have in common a loss of brain function that is usually progressive and eventually severe (Murphy 1986). There are over 100 different types of dementia, the most common being Alzheimer's disease, vascular dementia and dementia with Lewy bodies. Features of dementia include:

- loss of memory
- confusion
- problems with speech and understanding.

An individual may have more than one type and the age of onset can vary; however, it is generally more common in people over 65 years of age. Attitudes towards older people within our society are not always positive, and this may be echoed in the way in which people approach working with people with dementia. Some people believe it is an area of work offering few rewards and one that can be carried out by inexperienced, poorly paid and poorly motivated staff. People experiencing dementia may be frightened and behave in a way that causes concern to others and may have difficulty coming to terms with the changes in their mental capacity and well-being. Given the demands of working with people who have difficulty understanding what is going on around them, it is essential to have the necessary understanding, skills, training, creativity and commitment to meet these challenges (Gilloran & Downs 1997).

Although there are many different types of dementia, this chapter focuses on:

- Alzheimer's disease
- vascular dementia
- dementia with Lewy bodies
- fronto-temporal lobe dementia.

ALZHEIMER'S DISEASE

Alzheimer's disease is the most common form of dementia, affecting around 500,000 people in the UK, and accounts for approximately 55% of all cases of dementia (Alzheimer's Society 2006b). First described by the German neurologist Alois Alzheimer, it is a physical disease affecting the brain, which is irreversible. The changes result from 'plaques' and 'tangles', which develop in the structure of the brain, leading to the death of brain cells. The process begins in the hippocampus, the area of the brain associated with short-term memory. People with Alzheimer's have a shortage of some important chemicals in their brain that are involved with the transmission of messages within the brain (Thompson 1997).

Alzheimer's is a progressive disease, which means that gradually, over time, more parts of the brain are damaged. As this happens, the symptoms become more severe. The features of Alzheimer's include memory impairment, confusion and difficulty making decisions. At first, the changes may appear to be subtle but, even so, often cause concern for the individual. Other features include mood changes and social withdrawal, which could be associated with coming to terms with the initial features. As the disease progresses, people with Alzheimer's will need more support from those who care for them. This support should empower the individual to make decisions and choices as well as to ensure they are safe and cared for; eventually they will need help with all aspects of daily living (Hunter 1997).

Although there are some common features of Alzheimer's disease, it is important to remember that everyone is different. No two people with Alzheimer's will experience the disease in the same way, and all will need support that meets their own personal and cultural needs.

SOME CAUSES OF ALZHEIMER'S DISEASE

It is likely that a number of combined factors are responsible for Alzheimer's disease. These include:

- age
- genetic inheritance
- environmental factors
- diet
- overall general health.

Age is the greatest risk factor for dementia, but other factors are important. Although inherited factors may be a feature, they appear to be a less prominent feature generally, even if a parent or other close relative has the disease. This uncertainty is similar when considering environmental factors, and research continues. People with Down's syndrome who live into their 50s and 60s may develop Alzheimer's disease, and those who have had severe head or whiplash injuries appear to be at an increased risk of developing dementia. Research has also shown that people who smoke and those who have high blood pressure or high cholesterol levels increase their risk of developing Alzheimer's (Doll *et al.* 2000).

VASCULAR DEMENTIA

Vascular dementia is the second-most-common form of dementia and accounts for approximately 20% of all cases of dementia. It is caused by problems in the supply of blood to the brain (Cheston & Bender 1999). If the vascular system within the brain becomes damaged and blood cannot reach the brain cells, they will eventually die, which may lead to the onset of vascular dementia. A key feature of vascular dementia is the sudden onset (Alzheimer's Society 2006c).

There are a number of conditions which can cause or increase damage to the vascular system. These include high blood pressure, cardiac problems, high cholesterol and diabetes mellitus. It is therefore important that these conditions are identified and treated at the earliest opportunity.

Vascular dementia presents as stroke related dementia, small vessel disease related dementia and mixed dementia (vascular dementia and Alzheimer's disease).

Stroke related dementia can result from a single stroke (single infarct) or a series of small strokes (multi-infarct). A person may experience transient ischaemic attacks caused by stroke related dementia.

An infarct is an area of dead tissue, in this case, the brain cells. Multi-infarct dementia comes about when blockages in the blood supply to the brain occur frequently over a period of time in the smaller blood vessels in the brain, causing tiny areas of damage. The process and areas of damage vary, but tend to be gradual and widespread. The onset may not be noticeable at first, although with some people there may be a sudden change (Stroke Association 2006).

SMALL VESSEL DISEASE RELATED DEMENTIA

This type of dementia, also known as sub-cortical vascular dementia or, in a severe form, Binswanger's disease, is caused by damage to tiny blood vessels that lie deep in the brain. The symptoms develop more gradually and are often accompanied by problems with walking (Thompson 1997).

VASCULAR DEMENTIA AND ALZHEIMER'S DISEASE (MIXED DEMENTIA)

A diagnosis of mixed dementia means that Alzheimer's disease, as well as stroke or small vessel disease, may have caused damage to the brain.

Features of vascular dementia may be similar to Alzheimer's disease but depending on the type of vascular dementia, may appear in a different pattern.

Vascular dementia affects different people in different ways and the speed of progression varies from person to person. Some symptoms may be similar to those of other types of dementia but may include symptoms associated with strokes, such as physical weakness. The onset may be sudden and progress in steps, whereby an individual's condition may remain constant and then suddenly deteriorate following an infarct. In addition to features associated with dementia generally, a person with vascular dementia may experience epileptic seizures and periods of acute confusion.

Factors associated with an increased risk of developing vascular dementia include family history of vascular disease, medical history of stroke, high blood pressure, high cholesterol, diabetes (type 2), cardiac problems and sleep apnoea (Haran 2004).

Protection from vascular dementia can be increased by adopting a healthy lifestyle that includes a reduced fat diet, not smoking, moderate alcohol intake and seeking treatment for high blood pressure and diabetes. Men and people from Bangladeshi, Pakistani, Sri Lankan and Afro-Caribbean backgrounds are at higher risk of developing vascular dementia than other groups (Alzheimer's Society 2006c).

LEWY BODY DEMENTIA

Lewy body dementia was named in 1912 after the doctor who identified it. It accounts for approximately 15% of all cases of dementia. Lewy body dementia is also known as DLB (dementia with Lewy bodies), Lewy body, a variant of Alzheimer's disease, diffuse Lewy body disease, cortical Lewy body disease and senile dementia of the Lewy body type. Lewy bodies are tiny protein deposits found in nerve cells that affect the normal functioning of chemical messengers in the brain. Lewy bodies are also found in the brains of people with Parkinson's disease. The cause of Lewy bodies is as yet unclear (Lewy Body Dementia 2006).

Lewy body dementia is a progressive disease, with symptoms worsening over time, often over several years. People with this form of dementia will often have features of both Alzheimer's disease and Parkinson's disease. These features include memory impairment, disorientation and communication difficulties comparable to Alzheimer's disease and muscle stiffness, limb trembling and loss of facial expression (seen in Parkinson's disease).

In addition to these features, the symptoms and abilities of a person with Lewy body dementia may fluctuate by the hour. This leads to considerable distress for the individual and those around them, as it is difficult to explain and convince others that there is a problem. The Alzheimer's Society (2006a) suggests that other features experienced by people with Lewy body dementia include:

- clear, detailed visual hallucinations
- fainting or falls
- a tendency to fall asleep in the day and experience disturbed, sleepless nights.

The scenario below is an example of the way one person was affected by Lewy body dementia.

Scenario One

Miss M was 85 years of age and lived alone. She was diagnosed with Lewy body dementia following a series of investigations prompted by memory loss and disorientation accompanied by visual hallucinations of fish in her coal bunker. This led to her emptying the coal bunker and putting the coal in the sitting room. She also 'saw' children dancing in her garden. These episodes were not constant but were a very real experience.

She became worried about the children being out late in her garden and concerned about the fish having no water. Family members had difficulty understanding what was happening, especially as at times they would visit and she expressed no such concerns.

As with other forms of dementia, Lewy body dementia is more common in people over 65 years and affects men and women equally. Diagnosis can be difficult to establish as the features may be consistent with Alzheimer's disease or vascular dementia. However, visual hallucinations and trembling or stiffness in limbs should inform the diagnosis.

There are important considerations when treating people with Lewy body dementia. Neuroleptic drugs used to treat symptoms of severe mental health problems can worsen the Parkinson-type symptoms of someone with Lewy body dementia and may even lead to death (McKeith 1998).

FRONTO-TEMPORAL LOBE DEMENTIA

Fronto-temporal lobe dementia is a rare form of dementia accounting for approximately 5% of all dementias. It is more likely to affect people under 65 years, and affects both men and women. Causes of this type of dementia vary, with 50% of those developing it having a family history, which usually has a specific pattern associated with the progression of the disease. Causes for those with no family history are uncertain.

Pick's disease, dementia associated with motor neurone disease and fronto-lobe dementia is included in the term 'fronto-temporal dementia'. A specific feature is damage to the frontal lobe and/or the temporal parts of the brain, which are responsible for behaviour, language and emotional responses. This results in very different features from those expected in people diagnosed with the dementias mentioned above.

Most significant is that the memory remains intact but behaviour and personality change, with the individual acting in a disinhibited manner or being obsessive and rigid when previously they were outgoing and flexible. Adapting to these changes can be difficult and extremely distressing for the family and friends. The specific changes to personality and behaviour are different for each person affected by the dementia (Cheston & Bender 1999).

Language problems are a common feature in people with fronto-temporal lobe dementia. This includes difficulty in finding the right words, not speaking at all, using many words with very little meaning or content and a lack of spontaneous speech. Specific changes in eating habits may also occur, such as overeating or eating sweet things. As the condition progresses, the features resemble those of

Alzheimer's disease, with the individual requiring all their daily needs to be met by carers. It is important to recognise that these symptoms have a physical cause and cannot usually be controlled or contained by the person (Erb 1996). An example of a family's experience of Pick's disease is demonstrated in the scenario below.

Scenario Two

Mrs Collins was 63 when she was diagnosed with 'probable' Pick's disease. She was a widow and had four adult children, all of whom worked in the small town in which they lived. Although private, she was sociable and involved in the community.

The family became concerned when her behaviour and language changed. She became abusive and argumentative, and talked freely about sex, often asking intimate questions of friends and family. The family members reacted differently to the changes in their mother: some took offence at what she said; others looked for explanations and demonstrated concern towards her. There is evidence to suggest that Pick's disease has a genetic component, which left the family members with a number of questions and fears relating to their own future and that of their children.

MAKING A DIAGNOSIS

It is important to establish a diagnosis following a comprehensive assessment in all people with dementia, whatever the type. An assessment should lead to greater understanding of what the individual and their family may need or benefit from, and should assess skills and abilities and not purely determine loss of skills or level of disability (Cheston & Bender 1999). The process of diagnosing dementia and determining what type a person is experiencing is complex. It is necessary to establish a comprehensive family and medical history, along with changes in behaviour and health generally, both recently and over time. The symptoms and features of dementia may be exacerbated by underlying treatable medical conditions, such as:

- urinary tract and respiratory infections
- depression
- constipation
- thyroid or vitamin deficiencies.

It is beneficial to gather information from the individual and family members, and consent should be obtained from the person being assessed whenever possible. Time should be taken to explain things to the person with dementia, and information should be given in written and verbal forms (Miesen 1999).

A whole array of tests may be used, including:

- blood tests
- X-rays
- cognitive tests
- computerised tomography (CT) scans
- Magnetic resonance imaging (MRI) scans, which produce images of the brain showing the extent of any changes to the brain.

People with dementia are sometimes excluded from the process of diagnosis for fear that they will not cope and may become depressed or suicidal, although this is less usual than it used to be. Information and support are essential for the person receiving the diagnosis and the family. Many NHS Trusts have specialist memory clinics, which are specialist services providing assessment, diagnosis, treatment and support to people with dementia and their families (Alzheimer's Society 2006d). The scenario below provides an example of one couple's experience of receiving the diagnosis.

Scenario Three

Betty was keen that her husband was not told of his diagnosis as she feared 'it will finish him'. However, over time her husband repeatedly wanted to know what was wrong with him and became agitated and frequently angry. The secret became a wedge between him and Betty. It was the first secret they had had in their marriage of 55 years. Finally, Betty agreed to her husband being told, and the relief was apparent; they were immediately able to share the experience and deal with the situation as it was.

Early diagnosis may result in effective treatment to prevent or slow further deterioration in some types of dementia. It will also allow people to make informed choices about their future treatment and to be involved in any decision-making process. A comprehensive assessment will enable an informed diagnosis to be made, which is vital, because, as mentioned above, certain drugs that may be effective in treating symptoms in some types of dementia for some people may in fact make things worse for a person with another type of dementia (Greaves 2005). Drugs currently licensed for use in the treatment of Alzheimer's disease are:

- Aricept (donepezil hydrochloride; Eisai Pharmaceuticals, Teaneck, New Jersey)
- Exelon (rivastigmine; Novartis Pharmaceuticals, Basel, Switzerland)
- Ebixa (memantine; H Lundbeck A/S, Copenhagen, Denmark)
- Reminyl (galantamine; Shire Pharmaceuticals Group, Chineham, Hants., UK).

Only consultant physicians can prescribe these drugs, but GPs can write repeat prescriptions. There is currently no course of treatment to slow down the progression of fronto-temporal lobe dementia. Some drugs used in the treatment of people experiencing psychotic symptoms, such as hallucinations, may result in severe complications or even death in someone with Lewy body dementia, which reinforces the need for comprehensive assessment and diagnosis before prescribing medication for people with dementia (Alzheimer's Society 2003). A clearer diagnosis also means that the person with dementia and their carers will have an opportunity to access appropriate information on the condition, its likely progress and what can be done to manage the changes.

The use of drugs to control behaviour is not considered to be good practice unless all other avenues have been explored. This includes assessing physical needs, communication difficulties, distress and the person's need for time and understanding (Dempsey & Moore 2005).

COGNITIVE AND PSYCHOSOCIAL INTERVENTIONS

Any assessment or intervention should meet the needs of the individual and therefore take into consideration their cultural and spiritual needs and beliefs. Assumptions should not be made based on gender, colour, ethnicity, culture or disability, but should be tailored to the individual's needs and lifestyle. The client should be at the centre of the process and considered within the context of their social network.

Cognitive behavioural therapy is a recognised intervention when working with people with mental health problems but is not usually considered as an option for people with dementia. However, in the early stages of dementia, it can be beneficial in helping the client to develop more insight into the relationship between their thoughts, feelings and behaviour; it can also empower the client in having some control over their experience and to make sense of it all (Ashton 2003). Including people in the process of assessment, diagnosis and interventions can make the whole experience less frightening; however, people react differently and staff should respond to the individual and explore their expectations and beliefs about dementia.

Person-centred counselling can be beneficial to the client and carers, and recognising the impact of dementia on the whole family is a step towards working with them. Recognising each person's role and perspective within the family may give some indication as to what may be needed to support each member. Sometimes, friction will develop between family members as to what should be done, and because one person may feel they are doing most of the caring (Soliman 2003). The way in which the family members related to each other before the client developed dementia may impact on the experience of living with dementia. Although there are no cures for people with dementia, much can be done to support, empower and ease the symptoms and experience of living with the condition (Pusey 2003). Knowing more about the disease and understanding why the individual is behaving in certain ways may help him or her to cope with it. Speech and language therapists may be able to help with language problems – both understanding and expressing – and a multidisciplinary approach is advocated (see Chapter 14 of this book).

Carers and staff may be able to develop coping strategies, such as avoiding confrontation and working round obsessions rather than trying to change the behaviour of those affected. This can be done by responding to and exploring the feelings associated with the behaviour or what is being said. For instance, if someone is repeatedly asking to go home, talk about their home with them, find out what they like about their home, who lives there, what it feels like to be away from them and perhaps engage in some happy memories. This process is described by Seman (2003) as 'meaningful communication' that validates the person's feelings relating to what is being expressed through their behaviour or language.

Social interventions are important; opportunities for people to come together to share their experiences and to socialise in an environment where they are supported and not under stress to hide their difficulties can increase their self-esteem and confidence. Occupation is essential and can take a variety of forms. It is important that those involved in caring for and supporting the individual are creative and consider all sorts of things to engage and interest someone with dementia. Exploring their life story may give clues as to what may be of interest to them or spark some recognition and pleasure (Kitwood 1997).

When asked, people with dementia and their carers express a need for information. This should be available freely and in a language that can be easily understood. Understanding why the person may be behaving as they are can help carers to cope with the situation. It takes away a sense of blame or responsibility: it is the disease that is responsible not the person. Using different forms of communication is essential. Make use of touch, smell, music, images (especially photographs) and language, which are meaningful to the person with dementia. This can be done through finding out about their past and interests. Information about their childhood, work, favourite holidays, their own children and interests will provide a link and common focus for you and the client (Killick & Allan 2001).

Below are two scenarios that provide examples of how knowing something about a client's past can lead to a greater understanding of their current behaviour.

Scenario Four

Jim was 82 years old and had a diagnosis of vascular dementia. He spent a lot of time walking round the sitting room in the residential home he lived in, rubbing furniture with his hands in a very repetitive way. When staff talked to his wife about Jim's interests and occupation, it emerged that as a young man he had been an apprentice French polisher, something he loved. The war interrupted his apprenticeship. The staff gave Jim polish and cloths and encouraged him to polish when he wanted to. The change in Jim was amazing. He was more communicative, less restless and smiled a lot.

Scenario Five

Mrs Graham, 87, was a mother of nine and had many grandchildren. Being a mother was her identity and what gave her purpose. She was diagnosed with Alzheimer's disease. She could no longer carry out tasks independently and needed to be cared for throughout the day. She attended a day centre but did not engage in any of the activities and would repeatedly ask when she was going home; she said she was wasting her time there, doing nothing. The staff asked the family to provide them with a photo album of her family that they could look at with Mrs Collins. In addition, they collected some baby dolls and baby clothes that needed to be washed by hand. Mrs Graham enjoyed doing this and then dressed the dolls. The process of caring for something led to her feeling more settled in the day centre and encouraged her to engage with the staff, while doing something familiar and useful.

IMPACT ON THE INDIVIDUAL'S LIFE

Dementia undoubtedly affects an individual's life in just about every aspect. The impact begins as the changes start to take place. Forgetting things is a common experience and one that we all have, but forgetfulness associated with dementia is a very different experience, as the following scenario illustrates.

Scenario Six

Mr Owen was 74 years old. For as long as he could remember, he had been a perfectionist, with a keen eye for detail. He began to notice that he was unable to recall why he had entered a room. After making light of this and entering into a joke with his friends – 'I'd forget my head if it wasn't screwed on' – he was unable to get away from the feeling that something was wrong.

When he tried to discuss this with his wife, she reassured him that it was something that happened to her as well but Mr Owen knew it was different. Things continued to change for him, but he couldn't put his finger on just what was happening. Sometimes, he would forget there was anything wrong at all and would blame others for things he had done himself. He would become anxious and gradually withdrew from the social contacts he had always had. He and his wife began to argue, which led to more tension and worry for Mr Owen, although he would usually blame her for the disagreement. Any attempt to talk to Mr Owen about his difficulties led to denial or flippant explanations for his difficulties. Eventually, his wife spoke to the GP and Mr Owen was encouraged to make an appointment. The GP talked to Mr Owen about his difficulties and suggested he might have symptoms of dementia. Rather than despairing, Mr Owen was relieved that he 'wasn't going mad'. This was the first step to the couple having support for the changes they were both experiencing.

This experience is not unusual. Although some people may experience a great sense of despair, they should be supported by being given the opportunity to discuss their concerns and how their dementia may affect their life, and by being given information as to what help is available and by being involved in decisions about their care.

IMPACT ON THE FAMILY: QUALITY OF LIFE AS A CARER

The effect of dementia on family carers is well documented. The Admiral Nursing Service was established to work specifically with family carers of people with dementia. Their assessment schedule focuses not only on the client's needs but more significantly on those of the carer. This assessment includes the carer's mental and physical health needs, their need for support to continue being 'who they are', information, practical help and eventually letting go of their role as carer. Most people with dementia live in the community with about half of them being cared for by their family and friends, and the responsibility for caring usually rests on one person (Helmes *et al.* 2005). Although caring is recognised as being stressful, it can also be an opportunity for challenge and developing new skills, or learning that you can do more than you thought possible. The scenario below shows how one man felt that having the opportunity to care for his wife actually enriched his life.

Scenario Seven

Mr R, aged 81 years, cared for his wife, who had Alzheimer's and vascular dementia. He had been a successful businessman and described himself as 'arrogant and chauvinistic'. He expected his home to be run in a way that suited him with little regard for his wife's needs. When he became a carer, his life changed. He described the experience as 'a wonderful opportunity to be a better person'. He talked about the way he loved his wife and was glad to be able to care for her. His only regret was that it took her dementia to make him reassess his life and his behaviour. Other carers talk about having an opportunity to 'give something back'.

Reciprocity and mutuality are important aspects of being a carer (Motenko 1989). Caring can also have a negative impact on the carer's emotional and physical well-being. If the relationship prior to dementia affecting their lives was not good, maybe hostile or resentful, the experience for the carer may be very different – which will affect the person with dementia too.

The process of caring changes over time, just as the dementia develops. Carers may not see themselves in that role initially, and may not welcome it when they do. It is recognised that caring for someone with dementia can be more stressful than caring for someone with a physical illness. This is due in part to the changes in personality and the illness's impact on relationships. It is also something that can not be seen, but affects every aspect of life. The repeated questioning, anxiety and difficulty in accepting explanations takes its toll on the carer, who may experience frustration, depression and exhaustion (Nolan *et al.* 1996).

Carers describe how friends and family stop calling and social contact reduces. Families and friends experience a range of emotions and levels of understanding, which change as the dementia develops. Some families report feeling isolated and anxious, having gone through a process of change with the person they love. Sometimes, partners describe feeling robbed of the retirement they had looked forward to, and their adult children feel the loss of their parent while having to look after them. The way carers feel about their role depends on a number of factors, including the carer's personality and how skilled they feel in what they are doing. The more able, knowledgeable and confident carers feel, the more likely they are to report satisfaction in caring (Nolan *et al.* 1996).

This reinforces the need to work with carers and provide information and support to meet their needs. Carers are entitled to an assessment of their needs through the Carers (Recognition and Services) Act 1995 (Her Majesty's Stationery Office 1995), and more recent legislation, the Carers (Equal Opportunities) Act 2004 (Her Majesty's Stationery Office 2004), ensures leisure, work and education opportunities are considered within the assessment.

Care staff often comment on the responses of carers when a loved one is admitted to residential or nursing care, either on a long-term basis or for respite. Criticism over the way family carers complain about clothing, or that spectacles weren't clean are often valid, and may also be a way for the carer to express their difficulty in accepting that help is needed and that they cannot cope alone. Family carers want to be included in decision-making and involved in caring for their family member. They want to be respected not only for the role they have but also for who they are (Davies 2005).

The carer will have a wealth of information about the client and have a shared experience. Working as partners in care will benefit the client, their carer and staff because knowledge and expertise can be used to ensure the person with dementia receives the best possible care, and carers will feel included in the process. The person with dementia is more likely to maintain their identity and thereby feel less threatened and more in control of their life. The challenge to staff is to be flexible and open to establishing a culture of care that is empowering, supportive and meaningful to the client and carers, rather than an efficient, task-orientated regime.

This requires really knowing the clients and taking the time to find out what makes them who they are, even if the person is now severely affected by the dementing process. Taking time to preserve and value the identity of an individual creates an atmosphere of respect and person-centred care. Paying attention to cultural and religious beliefs honours the differences and individuality of the clients, and gives a message to carers that their loved one is in a place that is safe and respectful (Cantley & Wilson 2002).

MEETING CHALLENGES

Communication with people with dementia is often considered to be a challenge. Indeed, some people talk as though it is not possible for those in the later stages to communicate at all and that those in the earlier stages are unable to communicate meaningfully. It depends on what is considered to be communication. Verbal and non-verbal communications are crucial links between people and continue throughout life, even the apparent absence of communication tells a story – that of being ignored, neglected or unimportant. Goldsmith (1996) has written a lot about communication and asserts that not only is communication possible with people with dementia but it must be encouraged and facilitated. The first step in the process is to believe it is possible. It is necessary to engage with the person and interpret the meaning behind the words. To do so requires highly developed sensory acuity, the ability to engage with people using all our senses and to use our senses to express communication. Touch, tone, pitch and pace should be appropriate to the needs of the individual. To be unhurried and connect with the emotions being expressed will validate the person and their experience (Feil 1993). Attention to the environment is also necessary, trying to talk to someone in a noisy environment where there are many distractions may lead to confusion and anxiety. Good lighting will reduce the likelihood of misinterpreting visual images, and having space to walk around may make people feel less hemmed in. Other considerations include ensuring your posture and facial expressions are relaxed, allowing time for the person to process the information. It can take five times longer for a person with moderate dementia to process information, and even then they may have difficulty responding. Use short sentences with only one message and give time for a response before moving on. The use of visual images or objects can aid communication, for example when telling someone with dementia that they are being taken to the bathroom a picture of a bathroom may aid understanding and reduce anxiety. Underpinning all communication should be respect, genuineness, a desire to communicate effectively and a belief that it is possible (McCallion 1998).

Aggression often results because of poor or negative communication leading to confusion and even fear for staff and service users. Being sure that communication is carried out to meet the needs of the person with dementia reduces the incidence of aggressive outbursts considerably. Staff attitudes to aggressive behaviour reframe the experience, understanding it as a response to a frightening situation, frustration or panic, and may encourage staff to consider their own behaviour and approach, and to adapt it in order to meet the needs of the person with dementia (Miesen 1999).

'Wandering' is a term used to describe the apparent aimless walking observed in some people with dementia. This type of activity is rarely aimless. It may be an expression of frustration, boredom or restlessness and close observation may well give some insight into the cause of the behaviour. Staff need to have the capacity to cope with the behaviour and the skill to interpret the reason behind it to enable their response to be reassuring and meaningful to the person with dementia. Hussain (1982) found that 93% of all 'wandering' seemed to have a logical destination, with 53% of stops being within 1 foot of another person, and 29% being by an external view – both providing clear communication if only someone was listening. Aggressive outbursts are distressing, and every effort to address the cause should be explored; however, it should be recognised that anger is a natural response to fear, frustration and confinement.

CONCLUSION

The aim of this chapter was not to set out a list of rules and guidelines as to how to provide the best possible care for people with dementia but to encourage understanding of the experience of dementia and the need for person- and relationship-centred care. 'Relationship-centred care' refers to the importance of recognising the importance of relationships generally and the way in which they need to be considered when caring for people with dementia. This includes the relationship between staff and client, staff and family members and, of course, the relationships within families (Nolan *et al.* 2004). Staff need the attitude and skills required to work in such a way as to empower and include those affected in the process of diagnosis and care provision. This can only be achieved if they develop awareness of the effect changes in the brain due to dementia may have on the individual, and the impact upon their families.

Caring for people with dementia is a challenging and rewarding experience. To do so requires commitment and the highest level of skills in communication, along with an intrinsic belief in the right of people with this progressive, degenerative, organic brain disease to have understanding, human contact and support in order to experience this stage of their life with dignity, respect and compassion.

REFERENCES

Alzheimer's Society (2003) *Drug Treatments for Alzheimer's Disease: Aricept, Exelon, Reminyl and Ebixa*. London, Alzheimer's Society.

Alzheimer's Society (2006a) FactSheets, http://www.alzheimers.org.uk/facts_about_dementia /index.html, accessed 20 July 2006.

Alzheimer's Society (2006b) News and campaign, www.alzheimers.org.uk/News_and_ Campaign/Policy_Watch/demography.htm, accessed 21 July 2006.

Alzheimer's Society (2006c) Facts about dementia, http://www.alzheimers.org.uk/Facts_about_dementia/What_is_dementia/info_vascular.htm, accessed 20 July 2006.

Alzheimer's Society (2006d) Memory clinics, http://www.alzheimers.org.uk/swish.pl?query=memory+clinics, accessed 20 July 2006.

Ashton P (2003) Cognitive behavioural interventions in dementia. In Keady J, Clarke CL, Adams T (eds), *Community Mental Health Nursing and Dementia Care*. Maidenhead, Open University Press, pp. 88–103.

Bender M (1999) *Understanding Dementia*. London, Jessica Kingsley.

Cantley C, Wilson R (2002) *Put Yourself in My Place: Designing and Managing Care Homes for People with Dementia*. Bristol, The Policy Press.

Cheston R, Bender M (1999) *Understanding Dementia: The Man with the Worried Eyes*. London, Jessica Kingsley.

Davies J (2005) *Supporting Carers of People with Mental Health Problems*. London, Department of Health.

Dempsey OP, Moore H (2005) Psychotropic prescribing for older people in residential care in the UK: are guidelines being followed? *Primary Care and Community Psychiatry* 10(1): 13–18.

Doll R, Peto R, Boreham J, Sutherland I (2000) Smoking and dementia in male British doctors: prospective study. *British Medical Journal* 320(7242): 1097–1102.

Erb C (1996) *Losing Lou-Ann*. Brandon, VT, Holistic Education Press.

Feil N (1993) *The Validation Breakthrough*. Cleveland, OH, Health Professions Press.

Gilloran A, Downs M (1999) Issues of staffing and therapeutic care. In Miesen BHL, Jones GMM (eds), *Dementia in Close-Up*. London, Routledge.

Goldsmith M (1996) *Hearing the Voice of People with Dementia: Opportunities and Obstacles*. London, Jessica Kingsley.

Greaves I (2005) Improving practice. *Drugs in Context* 1(11): 31–39.

Haran C (2004) *The Diabetes–Dementia Link: Healing Well*. Philadelphia, Healthology Inc.

Helmes E, Green B, Osvaldo P (2005) Individual differences in the experience of burden in caring for relatives with dementia: role of personality and mastery. *Australasian Journal on Ageing* 24(4): 202–206.

Her Majesty's Stationery Office (1995) *Carers (Recognition and Services) Act 1995*. London, The Stationery Office.

Her Majesty's Stationery Office (2004) *Carers (Equal Opportunities) Act 2004*. London, The Stationery Office.

Hunter S (ed) (1997) *Dementia: Challenges and New Directions*. London, Jessica Kingsley.

Hussain R (1982) Stimulus control in the modification of problematic behaviour in elderly institutionalised patients. *International Journal of Behavioural Geriatrics* 1: 33–42.

Killick J, Allan K (2001) *Communication and the Care of People with Dementia*. Buckingham, Open University Press.

Kitwood T (1997) *Dementia Reconsidered*. Buckingham, Open University Press.

Lewy Body Dementia (2006) Toronto dementia, http://www.torontodementia.org/ related-Dementia_lewyBody.htm, accessed 20 July 2006.

McCallion P (1998) Maintaining communication. In Janiciki M, Dalton A (eds), *Dementia, Aging and Intellectual Disabilities*. Philadelphia, Brunner/Mazel.

McKeith I (1998) Dementia: drugs used for behaviour problems. http://www.alzheimers.org.uk/Caring_for_someone_with_dementia/Unusual_behaviour/advice_drugsbehaviour.htm, accessed 20 July 2006.

Miessen BML (1999) *Dementia in Close-up*. London, Routledge.

Motenko A (1989) The frustrations, gratifications and well-being of dementia caregivers. *Gerontologist* **29**(2): 166–172.

Murphy E (1986) *Dementia and Illness in the Old*. London, Papermac.

Nolan M, Grant G, Keady J (1996) *Understanding Family Care*. Buckingham, Open University Press.

Nolan M, Davies S, Brown J, Keady J, Nolan J (2004) Beyond person-centred care: a new vision for gerontological nursing. *Journal of Clinical Nursing* **13**(suppl 1): 45–53.

Pusey H (2003) Psychosocial interventions with family carers of people with dementia. In Keady J, Clarke CL, Adams T (eds), *Community Mental Health Nursing and Dementia Care*. Maidenhead, Open University Press, pp. 160–170.

Seman D. (2003) Meaningful communication throughout the journey. In Braudy Harris P (ed), *The Person with Alzheimer's Disease*. Baltimore, John Hoskins Press, pp. 134–149.

Soliman A (2003) Admiral nurses in community mental health nursing and dementia care. In Keady J, Clarke C, Adams T (eds) *Practice Perspectives*. Maidenhead, Open University Press, pp. 171–185.

Stroke Association (2006) What is a stroke?, http://www.stroke.org.uk/information/what_is_a_ stroke/common_symptoms.html, accessed 20 July 2006.

Thompson SBN (1997) *Dementia: A Guide for Health Care Professionals*. Basingstoke, Arena.

14 Therapeutic Interventions

S. LEE, A. EDMONDS AND C. HUBBARD

INTRODUCTION

The term 'therapeutic intervention' covers a range of treatments and activities aimed at enabling individuals to recover from a disorder or distress. The treatments and activities may have specific functions but each contributes to the overall well-being of the individual and that of the family, where appropriate. Therefore, no single treatment or activity can claim superiority or sole efficacy in the process of enabling individuals to recover.

Treatments and activities are delivered by different health care professionals or jointly, each having specific expertise and skills to offer. Increasingly, health and social care professionals (practitioners) share some common core expertise and skills. For example, family therapy may be delivered by practitioners who may be nurses, social workers (SWs), doctors (DRs), psychologists or occupational therapists (OTs). Hence, no one profession can claim the monopoly of expertise or skills in mental health (MH) care.

The term 'discipline' or 'professional' is usually employed to describe the practitioners. Each group has its own distinct education, which leads to a qualification that entitles an individual to practise within that profession. For example, music and drama therapists undergo preparation specific to their practice. The same applies to other professional groups. However, there are some elements within the different groups that are common. The teaching of communication skills features highly in the education of all professionals. It is the fusion of the expertise, specialist skills and attributes of the different professional groups that provides a holistic overview of the service user's condition, thus making the contribution of therapeutic interventions invaluable.

Prior to delivering therapeutic interventions in MH care, careful deliberations and considerations routinely take place by the multidisciplinary team (MDT), which is made up members of the different professional groups. While the professionals have the expertise and skills, engaging with the service user is the key to success in delivering meaningful interventions. Working in partnership with the service user and their family is essential before any decision is taken as to the appropriate intervention to be delivered. Family members are important partners in the care

Caring for Adults with Mental Health Problems   Edited by I. Peate and S. Chelvanayagam
© 2006 John Wiley & Sons, Ltd

ɔcess; they provide support to the service users round the clock and are under
ıtense pressure and stress themselves.

Options of therapeutic interventions depend on the nature and severity of the
mental disorder. It is therefore vital that individuals and families seek help early
so that the interventions required do not become too complex. The interventions
required may not involve admission to hospital and could be delivered as an out-
patient or at home. Interventions should integrate both health and social care needs
in order that a holistic perspective of the service user's position, in the context of
a family where relevant, is not compromised.

For the purpose of this chapter, therapeutic interventions may be categorised into
three groups:

1. activity-based interventions
2. psychotherapeutic interventions, including family work
3. physical treatments.

While it is beyond the remit of this chapter to provide full details for each
of the interventions, the following provides a brief overview of these therapeutic
interventions.

ACTIVITY-BASED INTERVENTIONS

Activity-based interventions cover a broad therapeutic spectrum. They range from
task-based activities, including those that have a social and communication aim to
those with a psychotherapeutic focus (Finlay 1997). Traditionally, these interventions have been provided by occupational therapists whose core skills lie in the
analysis and application of purposeful activity; however, many other professions
now contribute to activity-based treatments. Activity-based interventions can be
undertaken either on an individual basis or in a group.

The therapeutic aims of an activity can be diverse, for example with the activity
of baking the possible aims may be:

- to assess the level of function (cognitive skills), concentration, ability to follow
  instructions (verbal/written), sequencing skills, accuracy, timing, attention to
  safety, planning and organisation, decision-making
- to improve the level of function in any of the above skills through selection and
  grading of component tasks
- to improve confidence/self-esteem through the successful completion of a
  familiar task
- to learn new skills
- to encourage social interaction using a task-focused activity.

Given the range of therapeutic aims of an activity, it is essential that a comprehensive assessment of the client's needs is undertaken prior to participation in the activity to ensure that the chosen intervention is both appropriate and therapeutic. There follows a list of the most frequently used activity-based interventions in mental health services.

ACTIVITIES OF DAILY LIVING

This term refers to the range of activities undertaken by us all in our day-to-day lives. Attention is paid as to how a person copes with daily-life occupations in the areas of work, leisure and self-care. These activities are usually categorised under the following headings:

- mobility: the ability to move either independently or with assistance
- personal care: bathing, toileting, dressing and grooming, eating
- domestic care: menu-planning, budgeting, cognition, shopping, cooking, household chores including cleaning, laundry and basic home maintenance
- community skills: use transport, making appointments, paying bills
- leisure: interests and hobbies, social interaction, creative expression
- work/education/voluntary/carer for others: performance skills, concentration, tolerance, attention to detail and care in work.

Activities of daily living (ADLs) are used both as an assessment of functional level and as a treatment medium in both hospital and community settings. The ability to undertake ADLs is a significant indicator of mental and physical well-being and therefore contributes a vital aspect to mental health care and therapeutic interventions.

CREATIVE ACTIVITIES

Examples of frequently used creative activities include crafts, baking, writing, music and gardening. The therapeutic aims of these activities as with all activities as previously stated are numerous. They can include the learning of new skills and the experience of success and subsequent increased confidence through participation in and completion of a task. For some, the activity can provide an outlet for creativity and self-expression or may be seen as a possible leisure interest or hobby.

Creative activities are well suited to clients who have difficulty using verbally based treatment. McDermott (1988) researched the benefits of craft-based activity groups and found that there was a greater degree of interaction and positive communication in these groups than in those which were verbally based. As with all activity-based interventions, the activity chosen can be graded requiring more complex tasks to be undertaken by the service user, and the degree of support offered by the practitioner can be gradually withdrawn to encourage the development of greater self-reliance and confidence.

PHYSICAL GROUPS: SPORTS/RECREATIONAL GAMES

The psychological and physical benefits of remaining fit and active are well known (Moore & Bracegirdle 1994) and are therefore reflected in the choice of interventions for mental health service users. The range of sports used by mental health practitioners includes swimming, football, badminton, snooker, volley ball and air hockey. Increasingly, these activities when undertaken in an acute setting are linked to groups undertaken in local community facilities in order to promote social inclusion (Sainsbury Centre for Mental Health 2002).

The choice of activity will depend upon the desired therapeutic outcome. Team sports might encourage cooperation, tolerance, sharing, interaction and leadership skills. Games that include quizzes, board games and drama-type activities (e.g. charades) can also be used to encourage interaction and the use of cognitive skills. Any game or sport can provide the therapeutic experiences as indicated but can also give opportunities for enjoyment and the possibility of development as a leisure interest.

SOCIAL SKILLS TRAINING

The aim of social skills training is to help people to enter and be more effective in social situations. People who might benefit from this training may never have acquired the skills (e.g. people with learning disabilities) or lack confidence in their skills (e.g. anxious individuals). Trower *et al.* (1978) define those who might benefit from social skills training as those lacking the skills to affect the behaviour and feelings of others in a way that either they intend or society accepts.

A lack of social skills might be a primary source of stress leading to isolation and rejection, which in turn leads to mental distress and illness. Or it might be secondary to mental illness affecting social performance thus adding to the original source of stress. Social skills training is premised on the idea that skills are learnt and can be taught to those who lack them enabling them to learn new patterns of interpersonal behaviour that in turn will have a beneficial effect on an individual's mental health. Comprehensive training programmes such as those developed by Argyle and colleagues (Trower *et al.* 1978) will include both verbal and non-verbal skills. These skills are presented in sessions, with suggestions for training exercises for each. The suggested session layout is:

1. introductory skills
2. observational skills
3. listening skills
4. speaking skills
5. meshing skills
6. expression of attitudes
7. social routines
8. tactics and strategies
9. situation training.

Most social skills training programmes run as groups for a set number of sessions. Individual members will have specific goals to achieve over the course of the programme. A session's structure will usually include a review of the main points of the previous session and any homework assignments. Each session will have a particular theme and skill sequence, which will be discussed. Effective behaviour is modelled by the practitioner, which the service user can then imitate through role play. Feedback on the observed behaviour is provided to assist learning. A key feature of social skills training is the importance of putting into practice the skills learnt during the sessions and therefore the service user and practitioner agree specific tasks to try out between sessions.

ANXIETY MANAGEMENT TRAINING

The aim of anxiety management training is to equip a client with a range of coping skills to enable them to have greater control over the levels of anxiety they experience. Anxiety management training requires the client to be an active participant in their treatment, undertaking homework tasks, practising techniques and strategies. Training programmes using a cognitive behavioural approach have been found to be the most effective treatment approach (National Institute for Health and Clinical Excellence 2004b). Training can be undertaken on an individual or group basis. Group-based treatments are often undertaken as a closed-group course over six to ten sessions.

An anxiety management course will include the following elements:

* psycho-education: accurate information about anxiety
* skills acquisition: learning coping techniques and strategies
* application: putting training into action (Miller *et al.* 1981).

The interventions that are used to counter the components of the service user's spiral of anxiety are:

* *cognitive* (negative thoughts): education regarding the nature of anxiety and its different components and the anxiety spiral, cognitive restructuring to recognise, evaluate and modify anxious thoughts
* *behavioural* (avoidance of anxiety-provoking stimuli): systematic desensitisation and graded exposure to feared situations, role play and practising coping strategies for particular situations are helpful
* *physiological* (autonomic response): practise relaxation and breathing control; it includes techniques and encouragement to undertake relaxing activities (e.g. swimming, yoga, listening to music).

RELAXATION TRAINING

Relaxation training involves learning specific exercises and techniques to lessen both physical and mental tension. A range of relaxation techniques are used by mental health professionals and are taught on both an individual and group basis. The most widely used techniques can be categorised as follows (Keable 1985a, 1985b):

Physiological techniques

- progressive muscular relaxation (Jacobsen 1964)
- contrast muscular relaxation (Wolpe 1958)
- simple physiological relaxation (Mitchell 1977)
- biofeedback (Miller 1969)

Meditative techniques

- the relaxation response (Benson 1976)

Hypnotic/suggestive techniques

- autogenic training (Shultz & Luthe 1969)
- visualisation – guided/unguided

Modified Relaxation Techniques

- cue controlled relaxation (Cautela 1966)
- Alexander technique and differential relaxation.

ASSERTION TRAINING

Assertion training is a branch of social skills. Assertiveness is the ability to express feelings and ideas, both positive and negative, in an open, direct and honest manner while having consideration for the needs and views of others. Assertiveness skills training can be beneficial for a wide range of client groups, for example people who have difficulty in expressing themselves, experiencing anxiety, and having problems in managing their anger. Assertion training, as with other skills-based interventions, can be carried out either on an individual basis or as part of a group programme and will include active participation from the client in role play and homework tasks.

The content of training will usually include increasing understanding of the different communication styles – passive, assertive and aggressive. Attention is paid to recognising both the verbal and non-verbal behaviours in each communication style. Other areas covered will include a review of assertive rights (Smith 1975) and the range of assertion techniques, such as broken record (where the assertive statement is repeatedly stated), fogging (acknowledging that the other person has a right to their view) and discrepancy assertion (to clarify seemingly contradictory messages, for example to complete a report in a short time span and yet to make it as comprehensive as possible).

WORK/VOCATIONAL/EDUCATIONAL ACTIVITIES

The links between unemployment and mental illness are well documented and researched (Smith 1985). Work or productive activity that includes education and voluntary work provides an array of benefits from income, structure and enjoyment to a sense of identity and worth. Interventions that focus on work might include activities to increase skills related to work performance, such as:

- concentration
- time management
- social interaction
- assertion skills
- organisational skills.

Practitioners might liaise on behalf of the client to negotiate a gradual return to working hours or for an alteration in their workload, such as flexi-time.

For some mental health clients who have had difficulty sustaining or obtaining work, a vocational assessment is undertaken to identify interests and skills. Referrals to agencies that support and encourage people with mental health problems into work might be indicated. The client might then be offered the opportunity to be placed in open employment with support from an employment adviser. This is in line with the Government policy of social inclusion and has meant a move away from supported work schemes and sheltered workshops specifically designed for people with disabilities. Voluntary work is frequently recommended to clients as an initial step in working towards paid employment. Advice on the range of current supported work and training schemes and financial benefits are available from Disability Employment Advisers at local Job Centres, similar links can be made with schools and colleges to obtain student support services.

LEISURE ACTIVITIES

An important aspect of health and mental well-being is having a balance between work, leisure and ADLs. Leisure activities are those activities undertaken as a matter of choice and that are found to be pleasing and undertaken in free time. They can include entertainment, recreation, hobbies, sports, visiting and adult education, though this is not an exhaustive list.

Leisure activities can offer opportunity for social participation, creativity and growth in self-esteem and are therefore an important component of therapeutic interventions. Practitioners can encourage clients to maintain, resume or develop leisure interests as part of their recovery process. This might involve providing the opportunity for clients to undertake leisure activities while receiving acute care or supporting them to participate in unfamiliar activities in which there is the opportunity to learn new skills and discover interests to pursue in the community.

SOCIAL INTERVENTIONS

Historically, social interventions were undertaken by SWs but increasingly are now seen as an aspect of the care coordinator role undertaken by professionals from all backgrounds within the Care Programme Approach (Department of Health 1999) framework. Social interventions refer to assisting clients with their accommodation, employment, education and finances, social and family work. Having undertaken a comprehensive assessment of the client's needs; the MDT will work with the client in order to deliver the appropriate intervention. This might involve signposting a client to a particular organisation for further assistance, for example benefits advice, help with form filling, supporting an application to an agency and liaising with services or employers on the client's behalf.

It is expected that practitioners will have a good knowledge of the range of services and initiatives available to mental health clients, in order to assist them in accessing support and promote socially inclusive practice. The detrimental effects in respect to a lack of access to housing and employment on a vulnerable person, suggests the Social Exclusion Unit (2004), are:

- poverty
- reduced social networks and support
- a lack of social status and identity
- stigma
- physical health problems.

Schemes such as the Supporting People programme provide local authorities with money to finance a range of housing projects from 24-hour residential homes to one-hour-weekly floating-support schemes; similar projects are also offered by employment and education services (Sainsbury Centre for Mental Health 2004).

PSYCHOTHERAPEUTIC INTERVENTIONS

Psychotherapy is:

> essentially a conversation which involves listening to and talking with persons in trouble with the aim of helping individuals to understand and resolve their predicament. (Brown & Pedder 1991).

Therefore, on an informal level, it is something many people undertake at times with friends and family, and all care professionals engage in with their clients. On a formal level, it is a form of treatment by a professional with education in a psychotherapeutic intervention. Rather than treating the symptoms of the illness as the medical model does through the body, psychotherapy is 'concerned with the content of the symptoms and their meaning for the patient's life' (Frank 1995).

Psychotherapeutic interventions can help people understand their feelings and ways of coping in order to bring about change. The interventions might involve thinking about where these feelings and coping mechanisms come from, and trying to resolve past experiences and relationships that are affecting them, or they may focus on changing particular problematic thoughts and behaviours. For some people, psychotherapy can be instrumental in the resolution of their problems; for others, it can help in coming to terms with mental illness and the resulting change to life, and work on issues which trigger episodes and cause relapse. Psychotherapy covers a large group of therapeutic interventions; the most common can be divided into behavioural and psychodynamic therapies. A psychotherapeutic intervention may involve individual, group or family work.

Frank (1995) states that the shared characteristics of the different psychotherapeutic models are:

- the therapeutic relationship (i.e. the patient having confidence in the therapist as someone who understands, is knowledgeable and can help)
- a healing setting (i.e. a safe place, which reinforces the therapist's professionalism)
- a rationale (i.e. an explanation of the cause of the symptoms and a procedure for resolving them).

For out-patient psychotherapy, the client needs to be strong enough to cope with the feelings and memories that might arise from the therapy and the changes that they might realise they need to make to their lifestyle. In the Health Service, clients are likely to be offered therapy of between weekly and monthly frequency. They need to be able to manage those difficult feelings between sessions. Therefore, it is important for some people to have other support while in therapy, perhaps someone to be with after a difficult session or to see in between sessions, to help with practical problems or to monitor risk. This can help the therapeutic process as the client may find it safer to open up and use the therapy if they feel any difficult feelings can be managed. The length of treatment for psychotherapy will vary from a few sessions to a few years, depending on the needs of the individual, the type of therapy and the availability of services. Specialist in-patient units or therapeutic communities may offer more intensive and challenging therapy, as the client is in a supported environment and able to attend frequently. A few specialist organisations offer intensive out-patient therapy. Brief interventions may be offered at acute mental health admission wards, often as groups, and are aimed at a supportive rather than explorative level. They can also serve as an assessment for further therapy.

COGNITIVE AND BEHAVIOURAL THERAPIES

Behavioural therapy is the treatment of the symptom/behaviour. The argument for behavioural therapy is that 'it solves the problem without going into deep exploration of the problem or the history of the patient' (Wigram *et al.* 2002); therefore it is usually a short-term intervention of between ten and 24 sessions lasting an hour each. The most common forms of behavioural therapy in adult mental health today are cognitive behavioural therapy (CBT) and cognitive analytic therapy (CAT) (Ryle 1991). Both work on the theory that cognitions, that is thoughts and attitudes, are learnt and can be changed, which will consequently change the problem emotions and behaviours. So, rather than just changing a specific behaviour, CBT teaches the client to change their mental structure. The patient is supported to employ strategies to deal with the cognitions: distancing, distraction, challenging, building skills.

> Change is effected through new learning experiences that overpower previous forms of maladaptive learning and information processing. Change can be maintained over the long term as these newly acquired responses generalize across situations and time. (Hazlett-Stevens & Craske 2002)

CAT is newer than CBT. The main difference with CAT is that once the harmful cognitions have been identified any therapeutic method can be used to help the patient, and interpretations are made by the therapist. The cognitive therapies require the patient to be able to organise their thoughts and develop an understanding of the processes; therefore, they are not suitable for everyone. CBT has informed interventions such as anxiety management, which has been discussed elsewhere in this chapter.

PSYCHODYNAMIC PSYCHOTHERAPY

Psychodynamic psychotherapy has developed from Sigmund Freud and psycho-analysis. A central belief is that our early experiences and relationships affect how we function as adults, and that feelings, thoughts and experiences we cannot cope with (that we find unacceptable) we bury in our unconscious. This can result in conflict between the way we consciously try to deal with things and how we actually respond. We may become psychologically troubled and not know why.

In contrast to behavioural therapies, the aim of psychodynamic psychotherapy is for the client to increase their understanding of the cause of their problems, feelings and responses. For the client 'to identify and understand what is happening in his inner world, in relation to his background, upbringing, and development' (Brown & Pedder 1991). Change occurs through the person recognising the problems and the experiences that have contributed to their present state, resolution of issues from the past and the internal conflicts they have caused and reconciliation with the aspects of themselves they had found hard to accept. This happens on two levels. The client tells the therapist about their problems and experiences and the therapist helps them think what past experiences might be affecting how they respond to situations now, how they feel about these experiences and what they need to do to resolve them.

On another level is the notion of transference, which describes the feelings the patient (unconsciously) transfers onto others, based on values and opinions they have internalised from significant relationships as a child, usually the parental ones. The client acts towards others as if they were like the parent and interacts with them in a way that gets them to take on these attributes, for example being passive and eliciting dominance. The therapist, as receiver of these transferences, uses them in their work with the client on their client's current problems with relating: reflecting them back to the client, interpreting, sometimes holding them, until the therapist feels the client is ready to accept them, using them in how she relates to the client. For this to work, trust and confidentiality are important.

In group therapy, the group dynamic is important as a reflection of clients' relationships outside. As well as a forum to share problems and experiences with others that can empathise, it can enable clients to test their ways of relating by learning from others' reactions. Group psychotherapy requires a degree of robustness: the ability to accept feedback and not to worry excessively about the other members.

By its nature of exploration and development of the therapeutic relationship, psychodynamic psychotherapy is usually a long-term intervention; however, it is increasingly adapted for short-term treatment: short-term dynamic therapy (STDP).

THE ARTS THERAPIES

The arts therapies are forms of psychotherapy that involve creative ways to express and explore feelings and problems. This may involve a psychodynamic, behavioural or other theoretical approach but it is the use of the art form that is central. The core belief is that expression through the arts – visual, imaginative, sensory or physical – can enable expression of feelings and experiences that may be too difficult or too deeply buried to talk about. The art form brings another element into the therapy space, to help communication and reduce the intensity of the client–therapist relationship, making it more bearable. An arts therapy allows different levels of expression and exploration, which can be modified to individual need. This can be purely through the creative art being the medium with which to express feelings and problems, or time can be made for verbally reflecting on the connection between what has been created and the client's personal experiences.

Although many people can benefit from an arts therapy, it is often clients who have difficulty expressing themselves verbally, those who can talk for hours but not get to the bottom of the problem or those for whom talking about their experiences is too overwhelming who are referred for an arts therapy. There are four arts therapies:

- art therapy
- dramatherapy
- music therapy
- dance movement therapy.

Each therapy is different in what it offers the client and will appeal to different people. For example, a dramatherapy group encourages interaction and team work between members and so can help people work on their communication skills and ways of relating, while an art therapy group might allow clients to work individually while in the company of others, which can be all the contact some people can manage. There is no need to be accomplished at the art form to use an arts therapy: the emphasis is on the therapeutic process, not on the creation of a finished product. A willingness to try creative expression is important, and some anxiety is natural.

To practise as an arts therapist requires a specialist qualification at Master's level. Arts therapists may sometimes cofacilitate groups with other therapies or health professionals, or be assisted by support workers. They may supervise others running art-based groups, such as confidence through drama and creative art.

ART THERAPY/ART PSYCHOTHERAPY

Art therapy today is strongly influenced by psychodynamic psychotherapy. A non-directive approach is emphasised. In an art therapy session, the client uses the time to work on a piece of art of their choosing: painting, drawing or model making, for example. This may be a new piece each session or something they develop over time. The therapist and client may reflect together on the artwork, perhaps noticing the colours, textures and themes. If appropriate, interpretations are made and connections drawn to the client's feelings and problems. Seeing these visual expressions of their experience can help the client become more verbally articulate about them.

> Images arise from the patient's unconscious and contain conflict ... the assumption is that once these conflicts are made concrete they can be more easily understood (by patient and therapist), which in turn would assist in their resolution. (Naumburg 1958)

Sometimes, art therapy focuses purely on the art object as the container of emotions, and the therapist and client relate solely through the art. Transferences can be worked with indirectly through the art form. Groups may be 'open studio', where clients just work on their art as a form of expression, or more psycho-dynamic/analytical, where the time is divided between individual art making and talking together.

One advantage of art therapy is that interaction between therapist and client can be minimal, which can be more comfortable for some people. Another is that the artwork is visible and tangible: it can be kept and looked at again; change and development can be seen.

DRAMATHERAPY

Dramatherapy is by its nature a structured therapy and therapist-directive, suggesting activities and guiding the client through the creative process. Aids are provided for the drama, such as pictures, figures, small objects, stories and scripts, costumes and props. It may be particularly appropriate for clients who need the containment of structure and direction to feel secure. There are many possibilities to the drama from story-making to role play, depending on how imaginatively the client can work and what level of distance is needed from their problems. Dramatic distance is a central concept in dramatherapy. This is the distance between the drama created by the individual and their real life. The distance can be enhanced by using or creating stories about fictional characters that are not in the client's real world. It can enable personal material to be explored, through the drama, which otherwise may have been too difficult for the individual to address. Jones (1996) calls this process 'dramatic projection'. 'Clients project aspects of themselves into …dramatic materials or into enactment, and thereby externalise inner conflicts', which can then be worked through in the drama. The drama becomes a metaphor for the client's own experience. An example would be creating an imaginative story with picture cards, exploring what happens to the hero, what problems they encounter, how they deal with them, how they feel and exploring different endings. Through verbal reflection, connections may be made with the client's real life and new insights gained into how they feel, how they cope with problems and possible alternatives, or the exploration may stay in the drama and change might happen at an unconscious level.

For some people, using imagination is difficult, but they can use the drama in a more concrete way, for example creating a spectogram (Jennings 1986). This involves representing the important relationships in one's life with small figures and objects, experimenting with how they are arranged – who is in front, who is close or far away – and making connections between the qualities of the objects and who they are representing, for example a lion that is powerful and fierce because it is protecting its family. This work may develop into representing how life used to be and how the client would like it to be in the future and exploring what is in the way. In a group, clients can negotiate and explore group dramas and experiment with interaction and playing different roles.

MUSIC THERAPY

Music therapy often involves the therapist relating to the client through musical improvisation. The client will begin playing an instrument or making vocal sounds and the therapist joins them with an instrument they feel appropriate to the music. Techniques the therapist might employ include matching the client's expression, supporting, accompanying, empathising, creating boundaries and confronting. Transferences occur through the music and are returned the same way to the client, when the therapist feels they are ready to receive them, by the therapist making them audible. Therefore, there is close interaction between therapist and client and a relationship is created and developed through the music, but there need not be any talking. This can be particularly helpful for people with severe communication disturbances who have difficulty making emotional contact, with positive psychotic symptoms, with obsessive-compulsive symptoms and people who intellectualise (Wigram et al. 2002).

In group improvisation, the therapist may take more of a structuring and guiding role. Themes that music therapy can address include:

> intimacy/distance, aggression/non-aggression, dependence/independence, acting out/ emptiness, being present, disappearing, moving from one position to another, and creating boundaries/testing boundaries. (Wigram *et al.* 2002)

Other musical activities that might be used are performing pieces of music, composing and listening. Again, what is used will depend on the client and the aims of the therapy.

DANCE MOVEMENT THERAPY

In dance movement therapy (DMT), the therapist notices how the client is moving and can make interpretations or address through the movement work by physically making changes. Aims might be: reconnection to the physical self, improving interpersonal functioning and addressing emotional issues safely in a contained forum. Typically, a DMT session starts with a warm-up led by the therapist, then spontaneous movements from the client(s). In one-to-one work, the therapist might interact with the client's movements, in a similar way to the music therapist in music improvisation, mirroring, clarifying, elaborating, modifying – in essence, replicating the good mother–child relationship of holding, containing and synchronicity. This develops to the movements becoming more thoughtful and knowledgeable as their meaning is discovered: 'Some insight is gained into the impulses or feelings that might have led to that movement' (Stanton-Jones 1992). Then, if appropriate, this will be related to the client's life. A group might involve shared patient leadership and a less directive approach.

Essential to DMT are body language, body memory and movement metaphor. Body memory is the idea that we have developed, since early childhood, a motor response for every sensory input we have ever experienced; so we will react the same (physically) to new, similar experiences and yet may not know why they evoked that response. This suggests that our body may remember things our conscious mind has forgotten; so expression through movement can enable these memories and reactions to be worked with. The idea of movement metaphor is that a movement can encapsulate a symbol of unconscious expression that has meaning for the client. Meekums (2002) gives an example: 'A person may adopt a hunched posture when describing the "burden" they carry in life.' She gives an example of DMT with a man who felt he was spineless. She noticed he was moving only with his upper body as if broken off from his lower half. She worked with him physically on his coordination and balance until he was more able to deal with pressure. He was then able to make connections to his feeling and reflected that he now felt stronger (Meekums 2002).

FAMILY WORK

'Family work' refers to interventions when there is evidence of family dynamics related to, or impacting on, the problem for which the client has sought help. Broadly speaking, there are two different types of family work – family therapy and family interventions.

FAMILY THERAPY

Family therapy involves the treatment of the family as a unit, rather than dealing with the problem(s) of the individual member. The aim of the therapy is to reduce the symptoms in the person who presents with the problem (the client), by changing the way in which the family functions or its members relate to each other. This might be undertaken by redefining the problem as one which concerns the whole family rather than just the individual. A commonly used form of family therapy is based on systems theory. The family or system is viewed as being more than the sum of its constituent parts. The aim of the therapy is to identify and, if appropriate, change the way in which family members interact and communicate. This usually involves one or two practitioners meeting with the family on a regular basis for a number of sessions.

FAMILY INTERVENTIONS

Behavioural family interventions are one of a range of psychosocial interventions that have been found to be particularly effective in the reduction of relapse in those with a serious mental illness such as schizophrenia (Pharoah et al. 2003). The main goal of the intervention is to reduce the level of stress and expressed emotion in the family as this has been found to be a factor in relapse (Brown et al. 1972). The intervention is based on the stress-vulnerability model, which sees the client as being predisposed to developing illness at times of stress (Zubin and Spring 1977), and seeks to reduce stress within the family. This is achieved by a combination of psycho-education about the client's condition enabling the family to adjust their expectations as necessary and improve communication patterns. Practitioners work in pairs meeting with families on a regular basis; it is recommended that this should be for at least a nine-month period (National Institute for Health and Clinical Excellence 2002b).

PHYSICAL TREATMENT

THE HISTORY OF PHYSICAL TREATMENT

The history of physical treatment in mental health care settings can be argued as one of violent and unpleasant sufferings. Mentally ill patients were believed to have been possessed by devils or bewitched. Blood letting, purging, blistering and cold baths, for example, were often normal remedies as these interventions were thought to relieve madness. Manacles, shackles and restraint devices were commonly used to manage disturbed behaviour. For a detailed account of physical treatment in mental health care of the past see Fennell (1996), which traces the history of treatment of mental disorder over the last 150 years in the UK, and Jones (1993), which includes the treatment of mentally ill people in this revision of the history of mental health services; both are worthwhile texts. These texts provide an excellent historical overview of care and treatment that would bring the reader to the current trend in mental health care. Chapter One in this book on the history of psychiatry provides an account of how attitude and behaviour shaped the views of mental illness in the past.

However, developments in the passage of time (from the Victorian era) in the understanding of mental disorder or distress have changed radically. Present-day treatment options have also changed beyond recognition from the past. Insanity or madness is now defined in medical terms as mental illness. Since the early 1970s, the acceptance of mental illness into mainstream medicine has been symbolised by the presence of psychiatric wards in general hospitals.

PHYSICAL TREATMENT

Physical treatment implies interventions that are connected with the body rather than with emotions. There is a divergence of views as to the cause of mental disorder. One school of thought believes that it is a hereditary disorder of biological influence; the other, a psychosocial model, views it as involving maladaptive thinking or coping strategies leading to an inability to manage one's life or emotions. As a result, physical treatment may improve the mental condition but does not alter the service user's circumstances, which may require resolution in order that the individual maintains their overall well-being. Hence, a combination of physical treatment with other therapeutic interventions is indicated, and the contribution of an MDT is essential.

The main physical treatment option for mental illness is the use of medication. The groups of drugs are known as: antipsychotic, antidepressant, antimanic and anxiolytics. Electroconvulsive therapy (ECT) is an alternative to the use of medication in some cases of severe depression and psychosis. The use of these medical treatments is regulated through professional education and guidance on prescribing. On very rare occasions, neurosurgery is indicated in some extreme cases; its use is regulated by the Mental Health Act 1983.

THE USE OF MEDICATION

As a general rule, medication should only be given under supervision, monitoring and regular review. This is to ensure that the efficacy of the medication is maximised and the side effects managed. The individual's mental state should also be monitored so that the dosage of the medication can be adjusted accordingly. There is a need to work in partnership with the service user in respect of medication education so that the service user's views and belief systems are taken into account and that the treatment is managed appropriately and sensitively. Therapeutic intervention in the form of medication education empowers the user to actively participate and take control of their own treatment, leading to a better treatment outcome (Akerblad *et al.* 2003).

It is poor practice to continually prescribe any medication without regular monitoring and review. Some medications may have a toxic effect when the person does not tolerate the chemical or dosage given; this could have a negative or damaging effect on the person's well-being. Some medication requires regular blood tests to ensure that the therapeutic level is maintained. The National Institute for Health and Clinical Excellence (2002c, 2004a) provides guidelines on the use of some of the medication and also Healy (2005) has written an excellent textbook regarding the medications used in mental health practice.

Staff or carers involved in the administration of medication should inform the user of the side effects of the medication and how they may be managed. There are medications that may be given to counteract the side effects. Gaining the user's consent in accepting the medication is essential before the treatment begins, except in cases where the treatment is subject to Part IV of the Mental Health Act 1983. Treatment under the Mental Health Act is discussed in Chapter Six of this book.

Antipsychotic medication

The discovery of phenothiazines (a group of antipsychotic medication) in the 1950s transformed in-patient treatment and the lives of individuals. Although the medication enabled some patients to leave hospital with the symptoms of the illness significantly suppressed, the movement disorder caused by the medication was a prime concern. The long-term side effects of the movement disorder had been debilitating. There is ongoing research to further the development of antipsychotic medication that has maximum benefits and minimal side effects. Antipsychotic medications for the treatment of psychotic disorders are commonly termed 'neuroleptics', which may be given orally or by injections. Long-acting depot injections are given for maintenance therapy when compliance can be monitored more effectively. The slow-release property of the drug prolongs the desired effect. It has the advantage of the service user not having to take medication daily; the injection may be administered weekly, fortnightly or three- to four-weekly.

The purpose of the use of antipsychotic medication is to reduce or minimise acute psychotic symptoms and to maintain the long-term relapse prevention of psychosis (Ohlsen *et al.* 2003). Once the psychosis has subsided, medication enables the individual to have a more realistic dialogue with carers or professionals to formulate a plan of therapeutic interventions. Clearly, when a person's psychosis is eased, the dose can be reduced, but it requires monitoring so that relapses can be prevented.

Prescribing practice on the use of atypical antipsychotic medication was published by the National Institute for Health and Clinical Excellence (2002c).

In the 1990s, a new group of antipsychotic medication was introduced, they are generally known as the 'atypical' or 'second-generation antipsychotics'. These new antipsychotics are known for their reduced side effects, such as induced movement disorder. However, they have a tendency to cause a range of other undesirable side effects, such as weight gain, diabetes and cardiovascular disorder (Ohlsen *et al.* 2003). Staff involved in the administration of antipsychotic medication should determine whether it requires regular blood monitoring to ensure that the medication does not have an adverse effect on the white cell count; the user's cooperation and consent is essential. Clozapine is usually given to sufferers who are treatment-resistant, but unfortunately there is a risk that the drug may diminish the white cell count, which could be fatal if left unchecked.

Antipsychotic medication may be used to control behaviour that may place the persons or others at risk in acute psychosis. The key purpose associated with use that has a tranquilising effect is more common in hospital settings where the administration can be frequently monitored and reviewed for the management of violence or aggression. Its use is normally terminated or reduced when the acute phase of such behaviour subsides. The mode of administration may be given by mouth or injection. Anger management or relaxation training is an appropriate therapeutic intervention for those who have a propensity for such behaviour. De-escalation is also useful in preventing disturbed behaviour (Royal College of Psychiatrists 1998).

The term 'major tranquiliser' is often used to describe this group of powerful drugs. However, the *British National Formulary* (British Medical Association and Royal Pharmaceutical Society of Great Britain 2005) states that it is misleading to regard antipsychotics as 'merely tranquilisers' as they do not impair consciousness and that the tranquilising effect is of secondary importance in the treatment of psychosis.

Anxiolytic medication

Anxiolytics are effective in alleviating anxiety and anxiety-related disorders. People suffering from sleep, panic or anxiety disorders may find the use of this group of medication helpful in order to manage daily lives and the accompanied emotions of the disorder. However, their use in many stress-related disorders, for example unhappiness, may not be justified. Some users may become dependent on the use of anxiolytics; therefore, their use should not be long term and should be for the shortest possible duration. The continued use of anxiolytics as a coping mechanism should not be contemplated as a long-term solution; other therapeutic interventions such as anxiety management or learning coping strategies may be equally beneficial. The British Medical Association and Royal Pharmaceutical Society of Great Britain (2005) regards the term 'minor tranquilisers', which has been used to describe anxiolytics, as 'misleading' as 'their use is by no means minor' and that this group of medication differs 'markedly' from antipsychotics.

Antidepressant medication

The word 'antidepressant' implies an agent acting against depression; hence it is the treatment of choice for those with a diagnosis of depression. However, the National Institute for Health and Clinical Excellence (2004b) recommends antidepressants should not be used for people suffering from mild to moderate depression; therapeutic interventions should instead be considered. An atypical antidepressant of the selective serotonin reuptake inhibitor (SSRI) group should be used because it has fewer side effect than the traditional group of antidepressants known as 'tricyclics' (National Institute for Health and Clinical Excellence 2004a), and the service user is more likely to continue treatment. Further, for severe depression, the National Institute for Health and Clinical Excellence (2004a) recommends that a combination of CBT and antidepressant is beneficial.

Antimanic medication

The term 'antimanic' reflects the usage of this group of drugs. It is generally used for the treatment of mood disorders and maintenance to prevent relapses of mood swings. In acute phases of mania, antipsychotic medication may also be used to control the manic behaviour. Staff involved in the administration of antimanic medication should determine whether regular blood tests are needed to assess therapeutic levels, toxic effects and other induced disorders.

Electroconvulsive therapy

ECT, sometimes known as 'electric-shock treatment', has been available since the 1930s as a treatment option. Its use has always been controversial, and it is viewed as barbaric. How it precisely alters the brain's activities in alleviating mental disorder is unknown. The use of ECT is banned in some countries. In the UK, it is sometimes administered in a hospital setting to both in-patients and out-patients..

The user must consent to this physical form of treatment, except where Part IV of the Mental Health Act 1983 applies. It involves an electric current passing through the brain inducing a convulsion, following the administration of a general anaesthetic and a muscle relaxant. Following treatment, it is essential that the user is cared for as an unconscious person, with a clear airway ensured. Feeling confused is a common complaint from users for a short time when recovering from the treatment; supervision from staff is required.

A course of six to 12 treatments are usually prescribed and often given twice a week. It is recommended for sufferers of severe depression when medication has not proved beneficial. It is occasionally used for people suffering from psychotic disorders in circumstances when drug therapy has failed or is not suitable. Readers should consult the National Institute for Health and Clinical Excellence guidelines (2002a) for more detailed information.

Neurosurgery for mental disorder

The surgical procedure involves destroying brain tissue or destroying its function for the purpose of alleviating specific mental disorder. It is rarely performed but is still available to a minority of individuals suffering from very disabling mental illnesses when all interventions have not provided any relief (Royal College of Psychiatrists 2000). The surgery is carried out in highly specialist units, of which there are only a very small number in the UK. The Mental Health Act Commission (2003) reports a total of 13 referrals in the two years 2001–2003.

A referral is made to the Mental Health Act Commission when psychosurgery is indicated. A panel of three Commissioners visits the individual to ensure that provisions of section 57 of the Mental Health Act 1983 are observed before a certificate for the treatment is issued. The panel independently assesses if the individual is capable of consenting and agrees to the surgery and that the treatment should be given.

CONCLUSION

This chapter highlights the contributions of the MDT in therapeutic interventions from a health and social care perspective; and emphasises the importance of engaging and working in partnership with the service user and their family. There are different therapeutic interventions, as there are different clients with different needs, different ways of learning and different ways of expressing themselves. Applying a biological treatment model solely may impede the development of personal growth and realisation of the potential of the individual and their family. In promoting and enabling the service user and their family to learn to cope in their daily living, adopting an integrated and holistic influence in their care and with therapeutic interventions is critical. Given the unique membership of MDTs, where the different professionals deliberate on and think together about the expertise available within the team, enhancing the service user's and their family's qualities of life from an integrated health and social care perspective should be the norm.

REFERENCES

Akerblad AC, Bengtsson F, Ekselius L, von Knorring L (2003) Effects of an educational compliance enhancement programme and therapeutic drug monitoring on treatment adherence in depressed patients managed by general practitioners. *International Clinical Psychopharmacology* **18**(6): 347–54.

Benson H (1976) *The Relaxation Response*. London, Collins.

British Medical Association and Royal Pharmaceutical Society of Great Britain (2005) *British National Formulary 50*. London, British Medical Association and Royal Pharmaceutical Society of Great Britain.

Brown D, Pedder J (1991) *Introduction to Psychotherapy* (2nd edn.). London, Tavistock.

Brown GW, Birley JL, Wing JK (1972) Influence of family life on the course of schizophrenic disorders: a replication. *British Journal of Psychiatry* **121**(562): 241–258.

Cautela J (1966) A behaviour therapy approach to pervasive anxiety. *Behaviour Research Therapy* **4**(2): 99–111.

Department of Health (1999) *Effective Care Co-ordination in Mental Health Services: Modernising the Care Programme Approach: A Policy Booklet.* London, Department of Health.

Fennell P (1996) *Treatment Without Consent.* London, Routledge.

Finlay L (1997) *The Practice of Psychosocial Occupational Therapy* (2nd edn.). Cheltenham, Stanley Thornes.

Frank JD (1995) What is psychotherapy? In Bloch S (ed), *An Introduction to the Psychotherapies* (3rd edn.). Oxford, Oxford Medical Publications.

Hazlett-Stevens H, Craske MG (2002) Brief cognitive-behavioural therapy: definition and scientific foundations. In Bond FW, Dryden W (eds), *Handbook of Cognitive Behaviour Therapy.* Chichester, John Willey & Sons.

Healy D (2005) *Psychiatric Drugs Explained* (4th edn.). London, Churchill Livingstone.

Jacobsen E (1964) *Anxiety and Tension Control.* Philadelphia, JB Lippincott.

Jennings S (1986) *Creative Drama and Groupwork.* Bicester, Winslow Press.

Jones K (1993) *Asylums and After.* London, The Athlone Press.

Jones P (1996) *Drama as Therapy: Theatre as Living.* London, Routledge.

Keable D (1985a) Relaxation training techniques: a review (part 1). *British Journal of Occupational Therapy* **48**(4): 99–102.

Keable D (1985b) Relaxation training techniques: a review (part 2). *British Journal of Occupational Therapy* **48**(7): 201–204.

McDermott A (1988) The effect of three group formats on group interaction patterns. In Gibson D (ed), *Group Process and Structure in Psycho-Social Occupational Therapy.* New York, Haworth Press.

Meekums B (2002) Dance Movement Therapy: A Creative Psychotherapeutic Approach. London, SAGE.

Mental Health Act Commission (2003) *Tenth Biennial Report (2001–2003).* London, The Stationery Office.

Miller NE (1969) Learning of visceral and glandular responses. *Science* **163**(866): 434–45.

Miller RJ, Cullen B, O'Brien R (1981) Are you sitting comfortably? Psychological approaches to the management of stress and anxiety. *British Journal of Occupational Therapy* **44**(1): 5–9.

Mitchell L (1977) *Simple Relaxation.* London, John Murray.

Moore C, Bracegirdle H (6) (1994) The effects of a short term low intensity exercise programme on the psychological well being of a community dwelling of elderly women. *British Journal of Occupational Therapy* **57**(6): 213–216.

Naumburg M (1958) Cited in Waller D, Dalley T (1992) Art therapy: A theoretical perspective. In Waller D, Gilroy A (eds), *Art Therapy: A Handbook.* Buckingham, Open University Press.

National Institute for Health and Clinical Excellence (2002a) *Scope: Electroconvulsive Therapy (ECT) for Depressive Illness, Schizophrenia, and Mania.* London, National Institute for Health and Clinical Excellence.

National Institute for Health and Clinical Excellence (2002b) *National Institute for Health and Clinical Excellence Guideline on Core Interventions in the Treatment and Management of Schizophrenia in Primary and Secondary Care.* London, National Institute for Health and Clinical Excellence.

National Institute for Health and Clinical Excellence (2002c) *Guidance on the Use of Newer (Atypical) Antipsychotic Drugs for the Treatment of Schizophrenia: Technology Appraisal Guidance No. 43*. London, National Institute for Health and Clinical Excellence.

National Institute for Health and Clinical Excellence (2004a) *Depression: Management of Depression in Primary and Secondary Care*. London, National Institute for Health and Clinical Excellence.

National Institute for Health and Clinical Excellence (2004b) *Clinical Guideline 22 Anxiety: Management of Anxiety (Panic Disorder, with or without Agoraphobia, and Generalised Anxiety Disorder) in Adults in Primary, Secondary and Community Care*. London, National Institute for Health and Clinical Excellence.

Ohlsen R, Smith S, Taylor D, Pilowsky L (2003) *The Maudsley Antipsychotic Medication Review*. London, Martin Dunitz.

Pharoah FM, Rathone J, Mari JJ, Streiner D (2003) *Family Intervention for Schizophrenia*. The Cochrane Database of Systematic Reviews, Issue 3. Art. No.: CD000088.DOI:10.1002/14651858.CD000088. The Cochrane Library. Chichester, John Wiley & Sons.

Royal College of Psychiatrists (1998) *Management of Imminent Violence: Occasional Paper (OP) 41*. London, Royal College of Psychiatrists.

Royal College of Psychiatrists (2000) *Neuro-Surgery for Mental Disorder: Report from the Neuro-Surgery Working Group of the Royal College of Psychiatrists. Council Report (CR) 89, June*. London, Royal College of Psychiatrists.

Ryle A (1991) *Cognitive-analytic Therapy: Active Participation in Change: A New Intergration in Brief Therapy*. Chichester, John Wiley & Sons.

Sainsbury Centre for Mental Health (2002) *Working for Inclusion: Making Social Inclusion a Reality for People with Severe Mental Health Problems*. London, Sainsbury Centre for Mental Health.

Sainsbury Centre for Mental Health (2004) *Briefing Paper 26: The Supporting People Programme and Mental Health*. London, Sainsbury Centre for Mental Health.

Shultz JM, Luthe W (1969) *Autogenic Therapy (Vol. 1): Autogenic Methods*. New York, Grune & Stratton.

Smith M (1975) *When I Say No, I Feel Guilty*. New York, Bantam Books.

Smith R (1985) 'Bitterness, shame, emptiness, waste': an introduction to unemployment and health. *British Medical Journal* **291**(6501): 1024–1028.

Social Exclusion Unit (2004) *Mental Health and Social Exclusion: Social Exclusion Unit Report*. London, Office of the Deputy Prime Minister.

Stanton-Jones K (1992) *An Introduction to Dance Movement Therapy in Psychiatry*. London, Routledge.

Trower P, Bryant B, Argyle M (1978) *Social Skills and Mental Health*. London, Methuen.

Wigram T, Pedersen IN, Bonde LO (2002) *A Comprehensive Guide to Music Therapy*. London and Philadelphia, Jessica Kingsley.

Wolpe J (1958) *Psychotherapy by Reciprocal Inhibition*. Stanford, CA, Stanford University Press.

Zubin J, Spring B (1977) Vulnerability: a new view of schizophrenia. *Journal of Abnormal Psychology* **86**(2): 103–126.

Index

Caring for Adults with Mental Health Problems   Edited by I. Peate and S. Chelvanayagam
© 2006 John Wiley & Sons, Ltd